Complete Keto Air Fryer Diet Cookbook

Fit and Healthy Recipes to Enjoy your Meals

River Hunt

© **Copyright 2020 - All rights reserved.**

The content contained within this book may not be reproduced, duplicated or transmitted without direct written permission from the author or the publisher.

Under no circumstances will any blame or legal responsibility be held against the publisher, or author, for any damages, reparation, or monetary loss due to the information contained within this book. Either directly or indirectly.

Legal Notice:

This book is copyright protected. This book is only for personal use. You cannot amend, distribute, sell, use, quote or paraphrase any part, or the content within this book, without the consent of the author or publisher.

Disclaimer Notice:

Please note the information contained within this document is for educational and entertainment purposes only. All effort has been executed to present accurate, up to date, and reliable, complete information. No warranties of any kind are declared or implied. Readers acknowledge that the author is not engaging in the rendering of legal, financial, medical or professional advice. The content within this book has been derived from various sources. Please consult a licensed professional before attempting any techniques outlined in this book.

By reading this document, the reader agrees that under no circumstances is the author responsible for any losses, direct or indirect, which are incurred as a result of the use of information contained within this document, including, but not limited to, — errors, omissions, or inaccuracies.

Table of Contents

Baked Salmon & Carrot...9

Baked Shrimp Scampi..11

Tangy Salmon..13

Cheese Herb Salmon...15

Crispy Coconut Shrimp..17

Carrot Cake Cookies..19

Sun-Dried Tomatoes..22

Easy Apple Chips...24

Green Bean Chips..26

Snap Pea Chips..28

Crunchy Kale Chips..30

Dehydrated Okra...32

Lemon Slices..34

Eggplant Jerky...36

Curried Apple Chips...38

Delicious Cauliflower Popcorn.....................................40

Healthy Dehydrated Almonds.....................................42

Orange Slices...44

Dried Raspberries..46

Dehydrated Carrot Slices...48

Coconut Peanut Butter Balls 50
Spicy Rosemary Almonds 52
Lemon Avocado Chips 54
Smokey Tofu Jerky 56
Parmesan Zucchini Chips 58
Spicy Cauliflower Popcorn .... .60
Easy Kiwi Chips 62
Crunchy Broccoli Chips 64
Cabbage chips 66
Healthy Cucumber Chips 68
Beet Chips 70
Tasty Tomato Chips 72
Strawberry Chips 74
Smoky Eggplant Chips 76
Pear Chips .... .78
Broccoli Bites .... .80

Chili Lime Cauliflower Popcorn .... .82
Radish Chips .... .84
Dehydrated Bell Peppers .... .86
Brussels Sprout Chips .... .88
Dried Apricots .... .84
Parmesan Tomato Chips .... .86

Dehydrated Raspberries...88

Squash Chips..90

Lemon Chicken Jerky..92

Classic Cream Brùlé...94

White Chocolate Pudding..96

Cinnamon Grilled Pineapples..98

Tropical Pineapples Fritters...100

Apricot & Lemon Flapjacks..102

Baked Salmon & Carrots

Preparation Time:

10 minutes

Cooking Time:

20 minutes

Serve: 4

Ingredients:

1 lb salmon, cut into four pieces

2 tbsp olive oil

2 cups baby carrots

Salt

Directions:

1.Place salmon pieces in the baking dish. In a mixing bowl, toss together baby carrots and olive oil. Arrange carrot around the salmon.

2.Select Bake mode. Set time to 20 minutes and temperature 400 F then press START.

3.The air fryer display will prompt you to ADD FOOD once the temperature is reached then place the baking dish in the air fryer basket. Serve and enjoy.

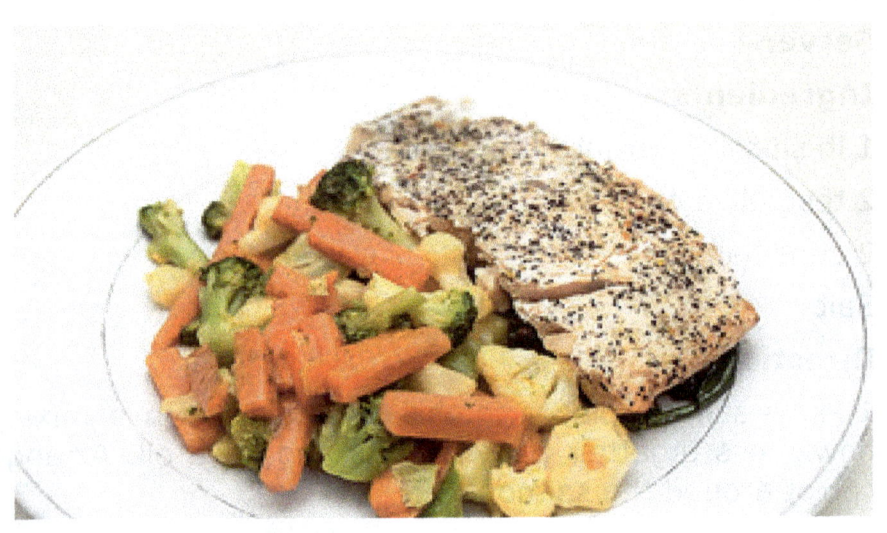

Baked Shrimp Scampi

Preparation Time:

10 minutes

Cooking Time:

13 minutes

Serve: 4

Ingredients:

1 lb shrimp, peeled and deveined

1/4 cup parmesan cheese, grated

8 garlic cloves, peeled

2 tbsp olive oil

1 fresh lemon, cut into wedges

Directions:

1. Add all ingredients except parmesan cheese into the mixing bowl and toss well. Transfer shrimp mixture into the baking dish.

2. Select Bake mode. Set time to 13 minutes and temperature 400 F then press START.

3. The air fryer display will prompt you to ADD FOOD once the temperature is reached then place the baking dish in the air fryer basket. Sprinkle with parmesan cheese and serve.

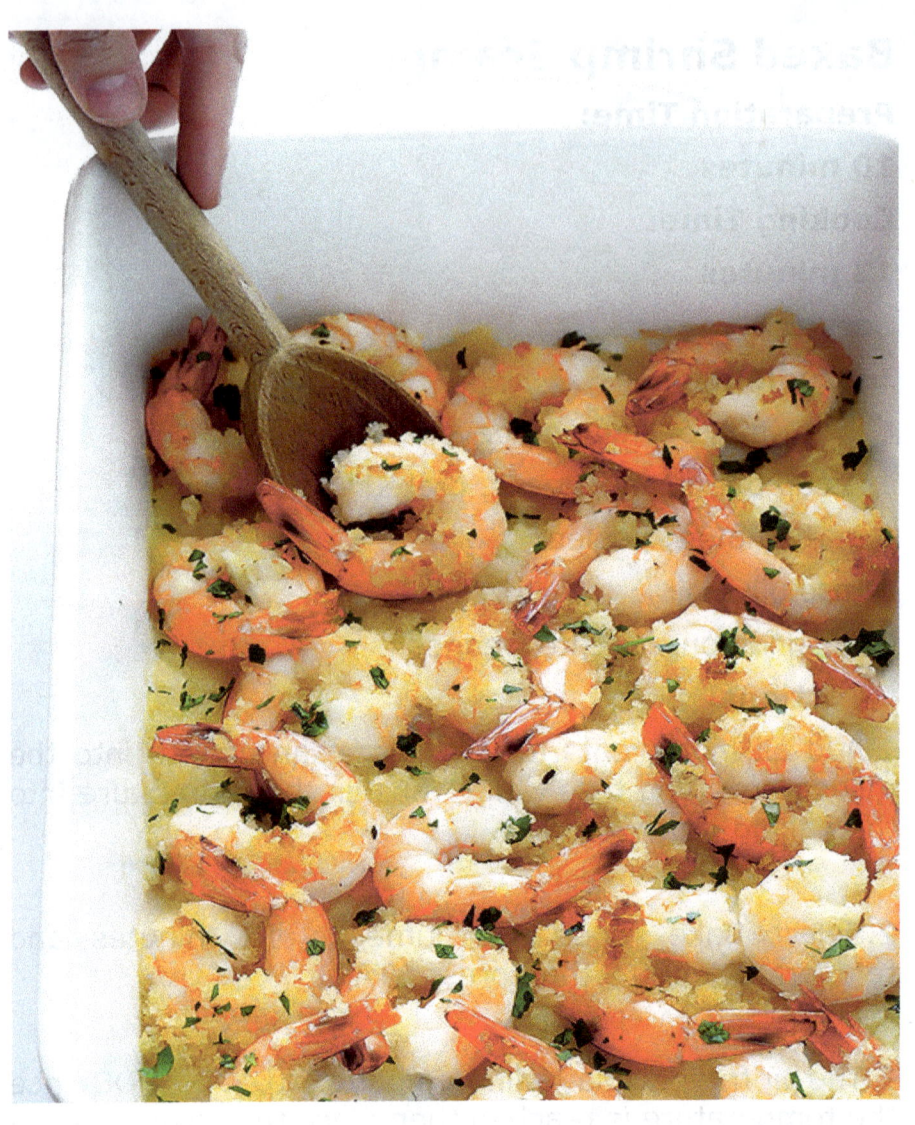

Tangy Salmon

Preparation Time:

10 minutes

Cooking Time:

22 minutes

Serve: 4

Ingredients:

2 lbs salmon fillet, skinless and boneless

1 tbsp olive oil

1/4 cup fresh dill

1 chili, sliced

2 fresh lemon juice

1 orange juice

Pepper Salt

Directions:

1. Place salmon fillet in a baking dish and drizzle with olive oil, lemon juice, and orange juice.

2. Sprinkle chili over the salmon and season with pepper and salt. Select Bake mode. Set time to 22 minutes and temperature 350 F then press START.

3. The air fryer display will prompt you to ADD FOOD once the temperature is reached then place the baking dish in the air fryer basket. Garnish with dill. Serve and enjoy.

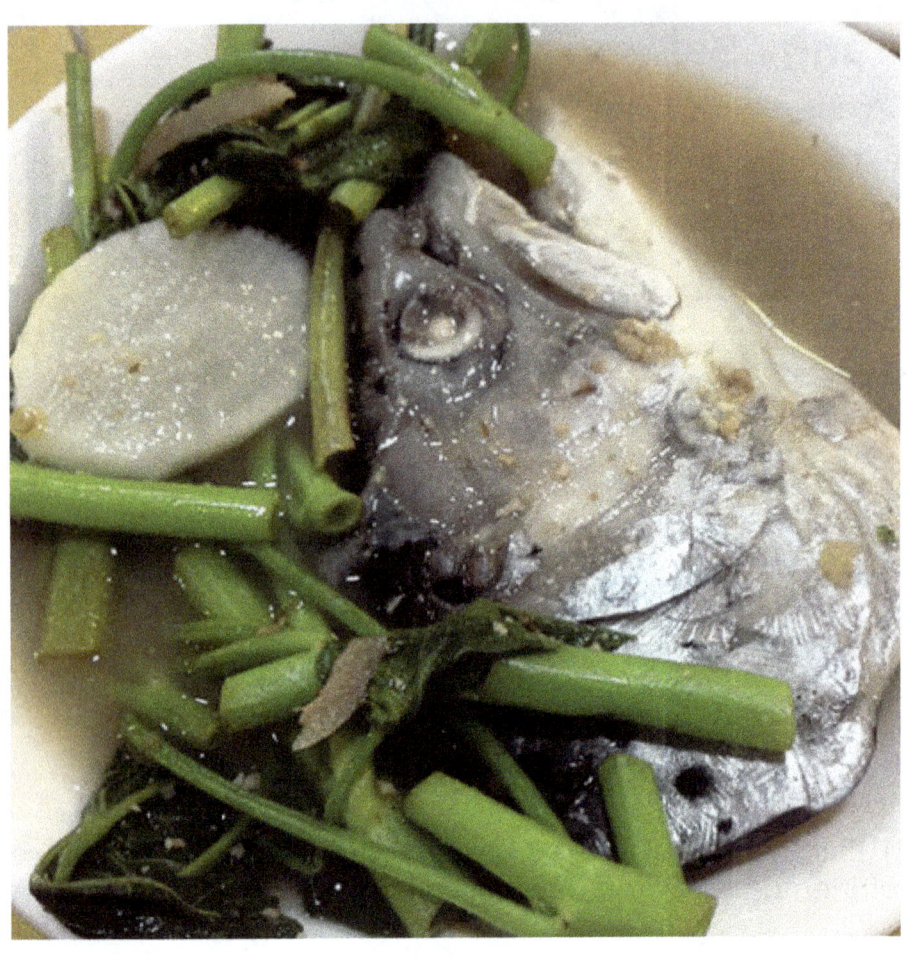

Cheese Herb Salmon

Preparation Time:

10 minutes

Cooking Time:

10 minutes

Serve: 5

Ingredients:

5 salmon fillets

1/4 cup fresh parsley, chopped

3 garlic cloves, minced

3/4 cup parmesan cheese, shredded

1 tsp McCormick's BBQ seasoning

1 tsp paprika

1 tbsp olive oil

Pepper Salt

Directions:

1. Add salmon, seasoning, and olive oil to the bowl and mix well.

2. Place salmon fillet into the baking dish. In a bowl, mix together cheese, garlic, and parsley. Sprinkle cheese mixture on top of salmon.

3. Select Air Fry mode. Set time to 10 minutes and temperature 400 F then press START.

3.The air fryer display will prompt you to ADD FOOD once the temperature is reached then place the baking dish in the air fryer basket. Serve and enjoy.

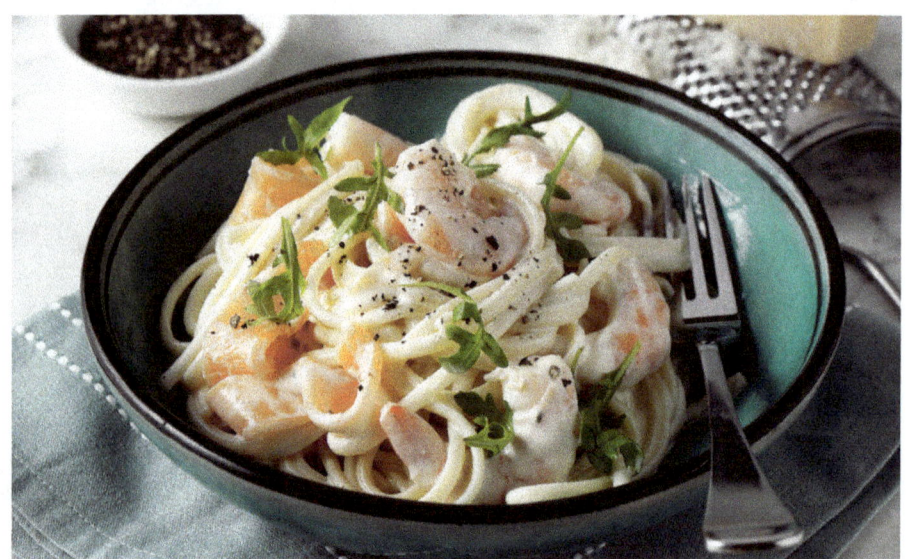

Crispy Coconut Shrimp

Preparation Time:

10 minutes

Cooking Time:

5 minutes

Serve: 4

Ingredients:

2 egg whites

16 oz shrimp, peeled

1/2 cup shredded coconut

1/2 cup almond flour

1/2 tsp salt

Directions:

1. Whisk egg whites in a shallow dish. In a bowl, mix together shredded coconut and almond flour.

2. Dip shrimp into the egg then coat with coconut mixture. Select Air Fry mode.

3. Set time to 5 minutes and temperature 400 F then press START.

4. The air fryer display will prompt you to ADD FOOD once the temperature is reached then place coated shrimp in the air fryer basket. Serve and enjoy.

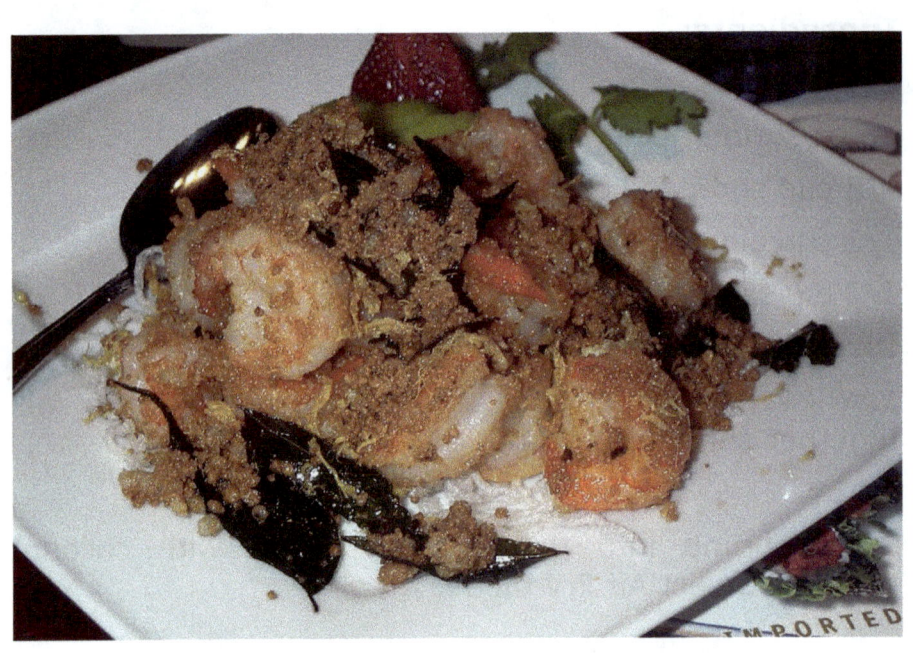

Carrot Cake Cookies

Preparation Time:

10 minutes

Cooking Time:

4 hours

Serve: 20

Ingredients:

2 cups carrots, grated

2 cups almond flour

1/8 tsp nutmeg

1/8 tsp allspice

1/8 tsp cloves

1/2 tsp cinnamon

6 tbsp unsweetened coconut milk

15 drops liquid stevia

1 tsp vanilla

Directions:

1. In a bowl, mix together almond flour, nutmeg, allspice, cloves, and cinnamon.

2. Add grated carrots, coconut milk, vanilla, and stevia and mix until well combined.

3. Place the cooking tray in the air fryer basket. Place piece of parchment paper into the air fryer basket.

4.Make small cookies from mixture and place in the air fryer basket. Select Dehydrate mode.

5.Set time to 4 hours and temperature 125 F then press START. Store in an airtight container.

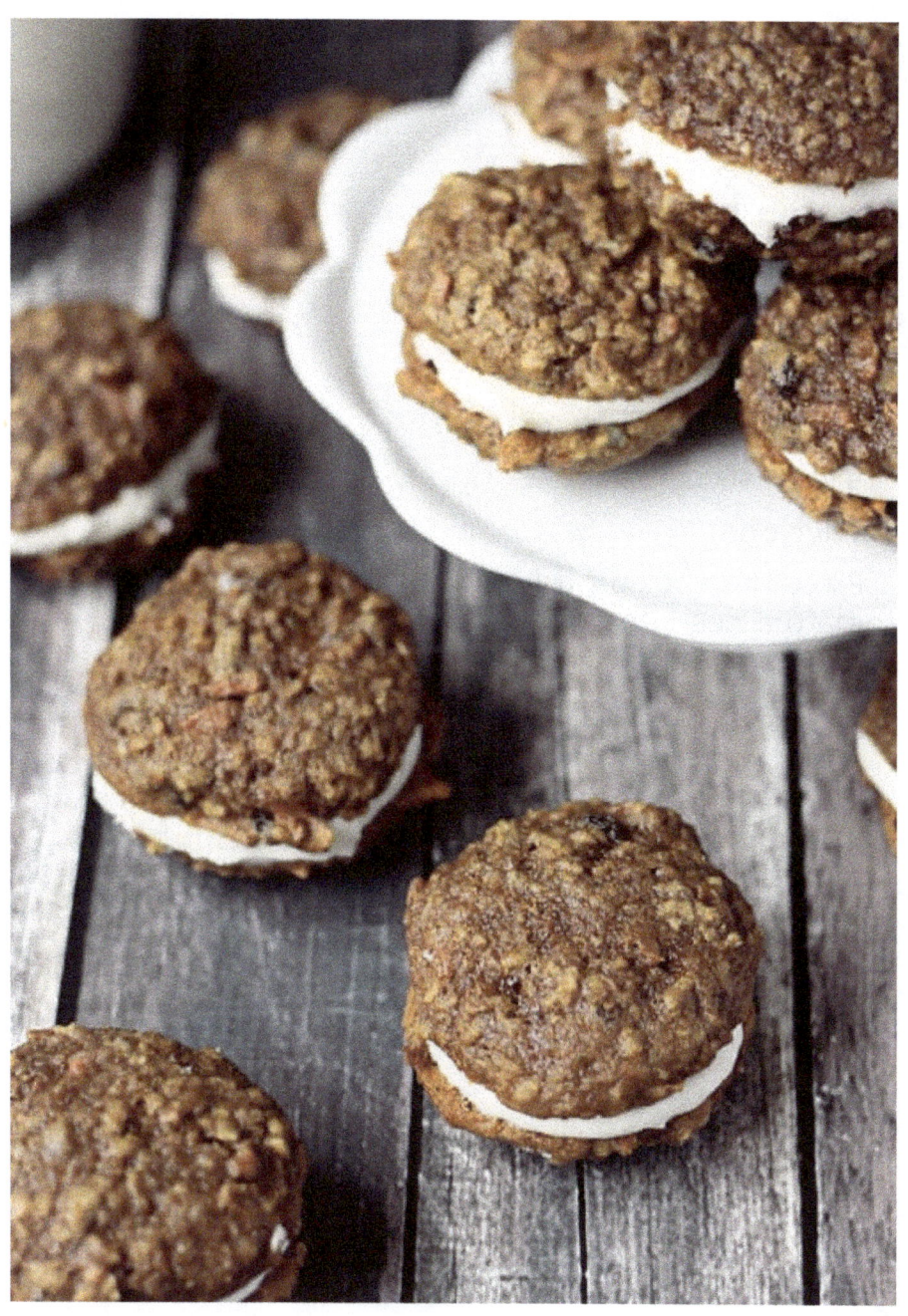

Sun-Dried Tomatoes

Preparation Time:

10 minutes

Cooking Time:

12 hours

Serve: 4

Ingredients:

2 lbs fresh tomatoes, cut into

1/4-inch slices Salt

Directions:

1. Place the cooking tray in the air fryer basket. Arrange tomato slices into the air fryer basket.

2. Select Dehydrate mode. Set time to 6-12 hours and temperature 145 F then press START. Store in an airtight container.

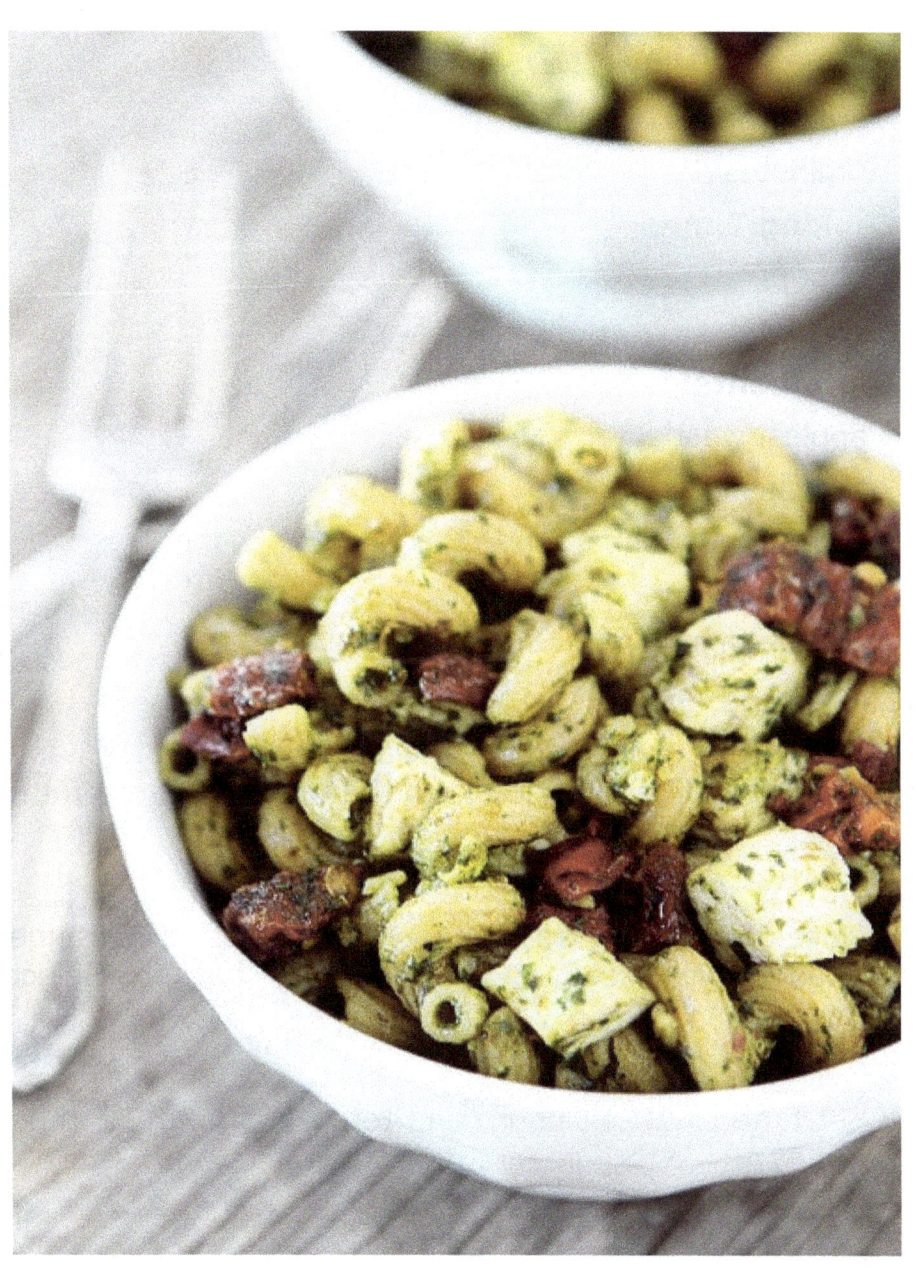

Easy Apple Chips

Preparation Time:

10 minutes

Cooking Time:

12 hours

Serve: 4

Ingredients:

3 apples, washed and cut into

3/8-inch slices

1 tbsp ground cinnamon

2 tbsp fresh lemon juice

2 cups of water

Directions:

1. In a bowl, mix together water, lemon juice, and cinnamon. Add apple slices into the water and soak for 8 hours.

2. Place the cooking tray in the air fryer basket. Arrange soaked apple slices in the air fryer basket. Select Dehydrate mode.

3. Set time to 10-12 hours and temperature 145 F then press START. Store in an airtight container.

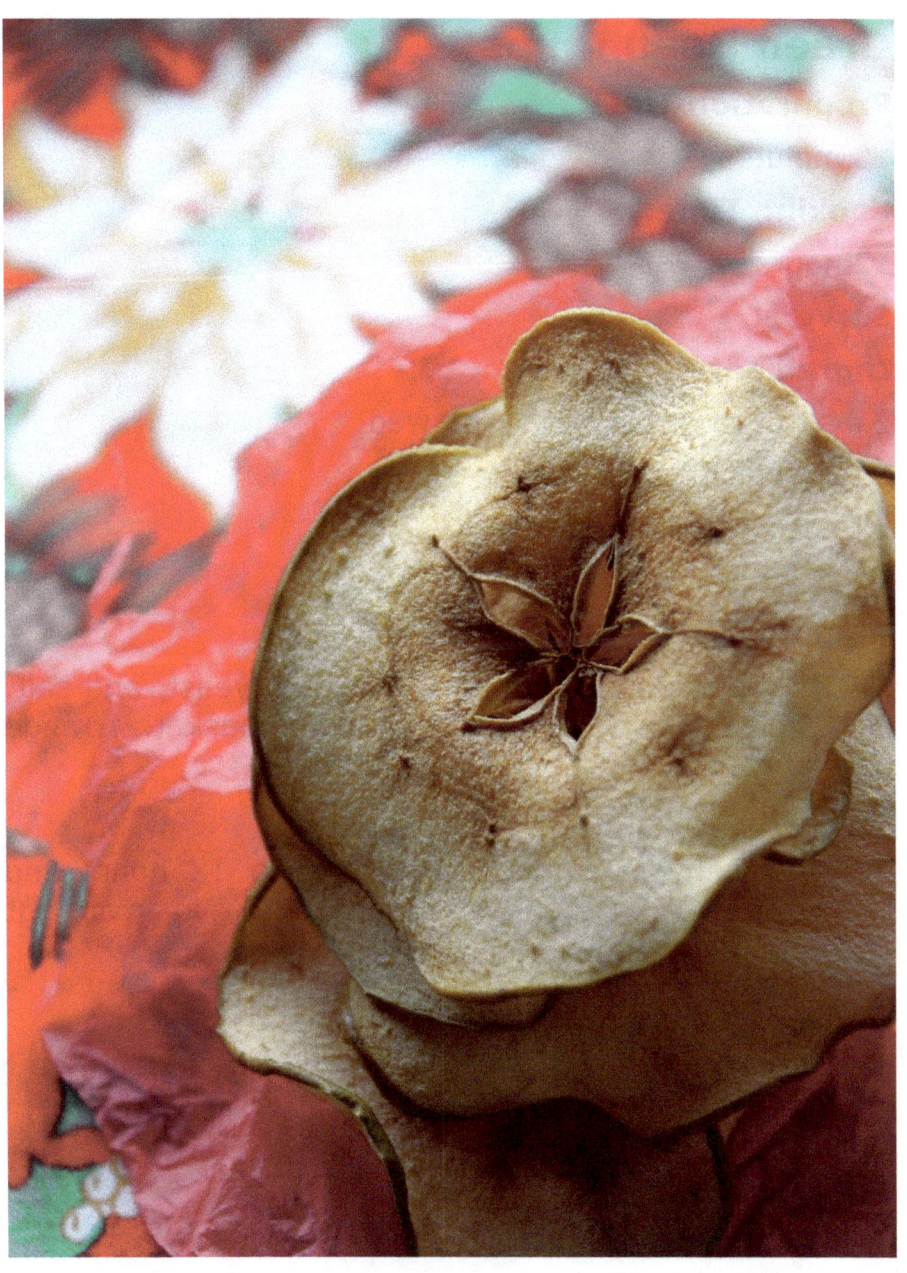

Green Bean Chips

Preparation Time:

10 minutes

Cooking Time:

12 hours

Serve: 4

Ingredients:

2 lbs frozen green beans, thawed

2 tbsp nutritional yeast

2 tbsp coconut oil, melted

1 1/2 tsp salt

Directions:

1.Toss green beans with oil, nutritional yeast, and salt. Place the cooking tray in the air fryer basket. Arrange green beans in the air fryer basket.

2.Select Dehydrate mode. Set time to 12 hours and temperature 125 F then press START. Store in an airtight container.

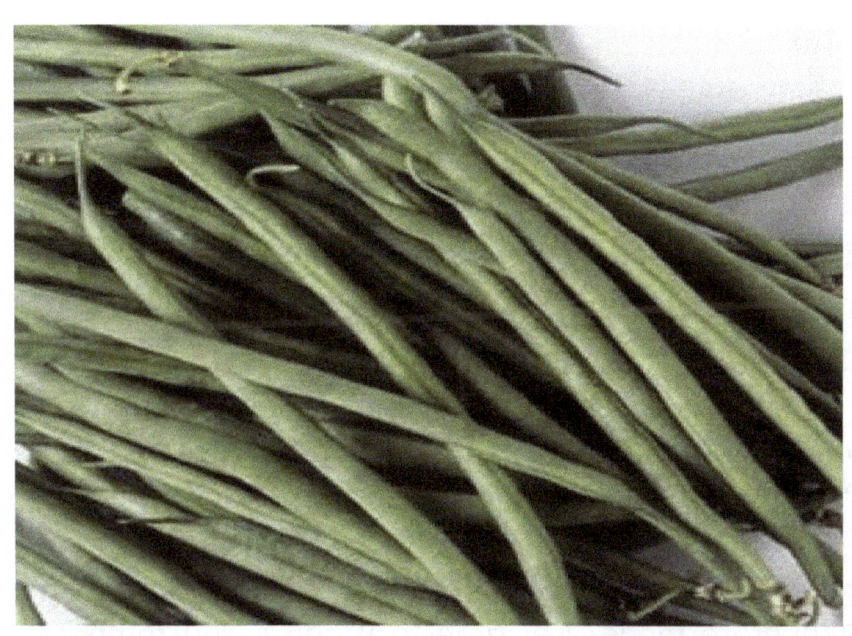

Snap Pea Chips

Preparation Time:

10 minutes

Cooking Time:

8 hours

Serve: 6

Ingredients:

3 cups snap peas

2 tbsp olive oil

1/2 tsp garlic powder

2 tbsp nutritional yeast

1/2 tsp sea salt

Directions:

1. Toss snap peas with oil, garlic powder, nutritional yeast, and salt. Place the cooking tray in the air fryer basket.

2. Arrange snap peas in the air fryer basket. Select Dehydrate mode. Set time to 8 hours and temperature 135 F then press START.

3. Store in an airtight container.

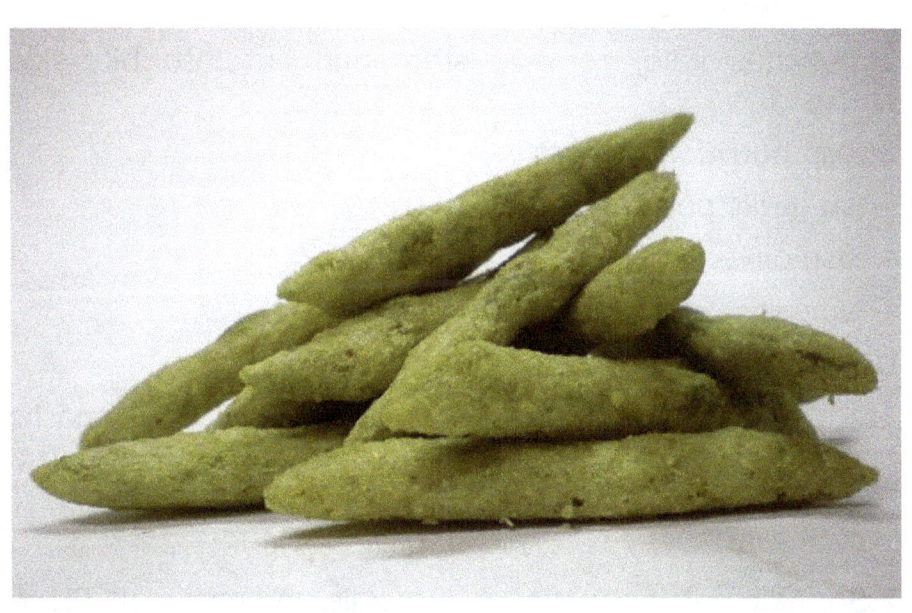

Crunchy Kale Chips

Preparation Time:

10 minutes

Cooking Time:

2 hours

Serve: 4

Ingredients:

2 bunches kale, remove stem and cut into bite-size pieces

3 tbsp nutritional yeast

2 tsp garlic powder

1 tbsp olive oil

1 tsp salt

Directions:

1. Add kale pieces into the mixing bowl. Add garlic powder, oil, and salt over kale and massage into the leaves.

2. Sprinkle nutritional yeast over kale and toss well. Place the cooking tray in the air fryer basket. Arrange kale in the air fryer basket.

3. Select Dehydrate mode. Set time to 2 hours and temperature 160 F then press START. Store in an airtight container.

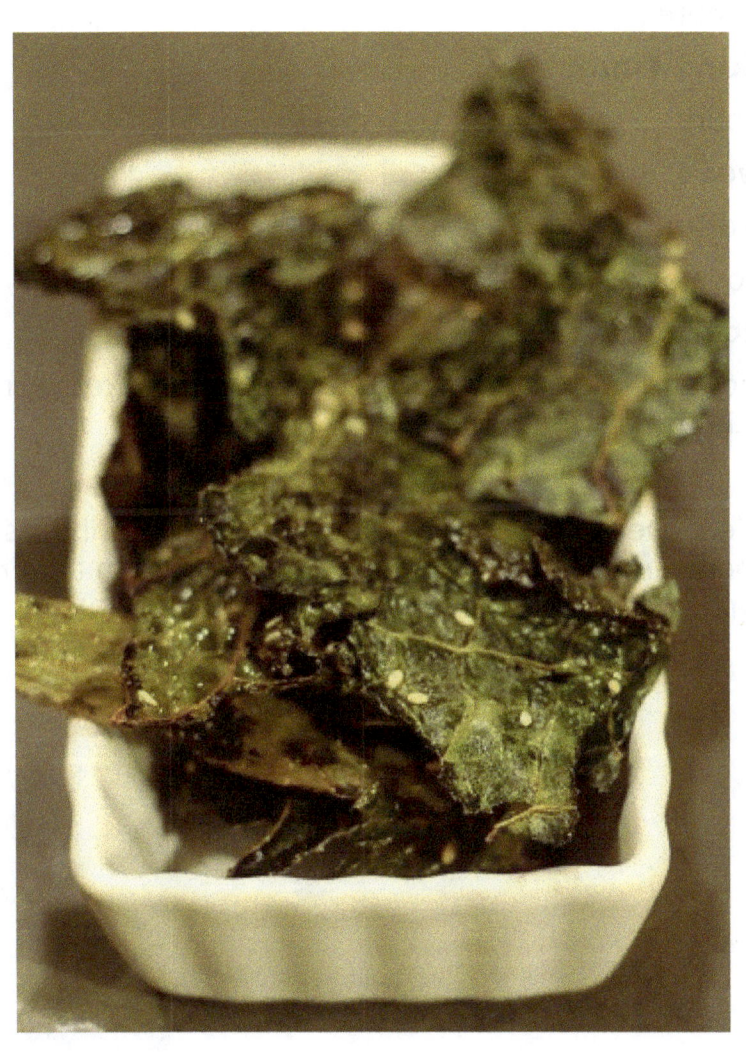

Dehydrated Okra

Preparation Time:

10 minutes

Cooking Time:

24 hours

Serve: 4

Ingredients:

12 pods okra, slice into rounds

Directions:

1. Place the cooking tray in the air fryer basket. Arrange okra in the air fryer basket.

2. Select Dehydrate mode. Set time to 24 hours and temperature 130 F then press START. Store in an airtight container.

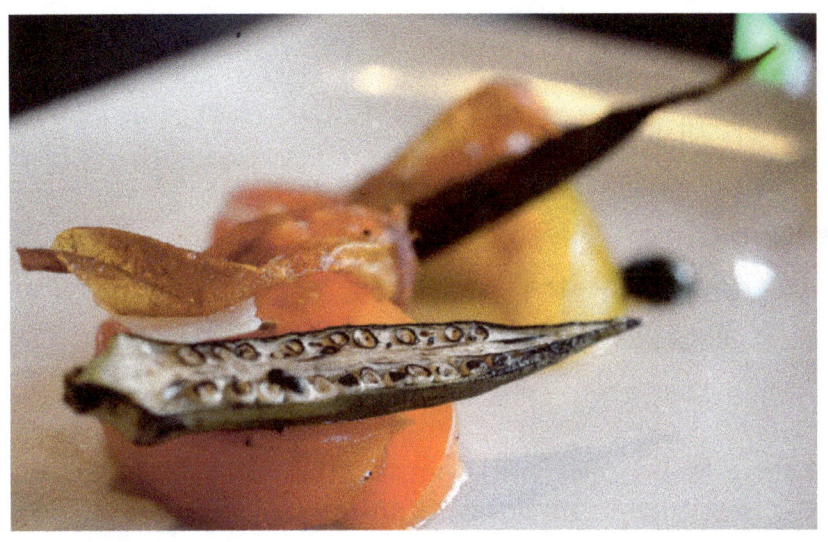

Lemon Slices

Preparation Time:

10 minutes

Cooking Time:

5 hours

Serve: 6

Ingredients:

4 lemons, cut into

1/4-inch thick slices

Directions:

1. Place the cooking tray in the air fryer basket. Arrange lemon slices in the air fryer basket. Select Dehydrate mode.

2. Set time to 5 hours and temperature 170 F then press START. Store in an airtight container.

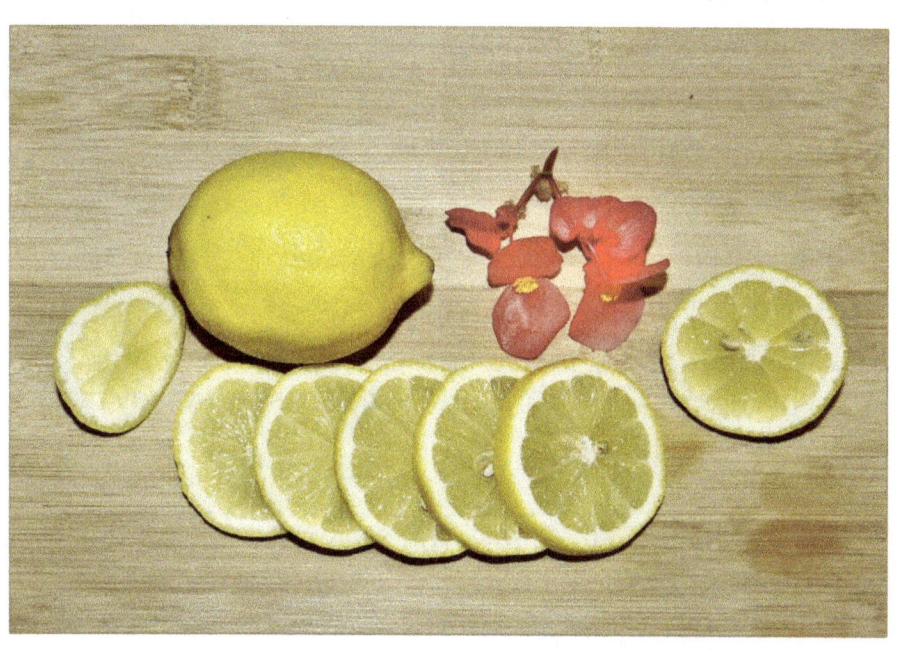

Eggplant Jerky

Preparation Time:

10 minutes

Cooking Time:

10 hours

Serve: 3

Ingredients:

2 medium eggplant, cut into

1/4-inch thick slices

1/2 tsp red chili flakes

3 tbsp soy sauce

2 tbsp water

Directions:

1. In a small bowl, mix together soy sauce, water, and red chili flakes. Brush eggplant slices with soy sauce mixture.

2. Place eggplant slices into the dish, cover, and place in the refrigerator for 2 hours.

3. Place the cooking tray in the air fryer basket. Place piece of parchment paper into the air fryer basket.

4. Arrange eggplant slices onto the parchment paper in the air fryer basket.

5.Select Dehydrate mode. Set time to 10 hours and temperature 115 F then press START. Store in an airtight container.

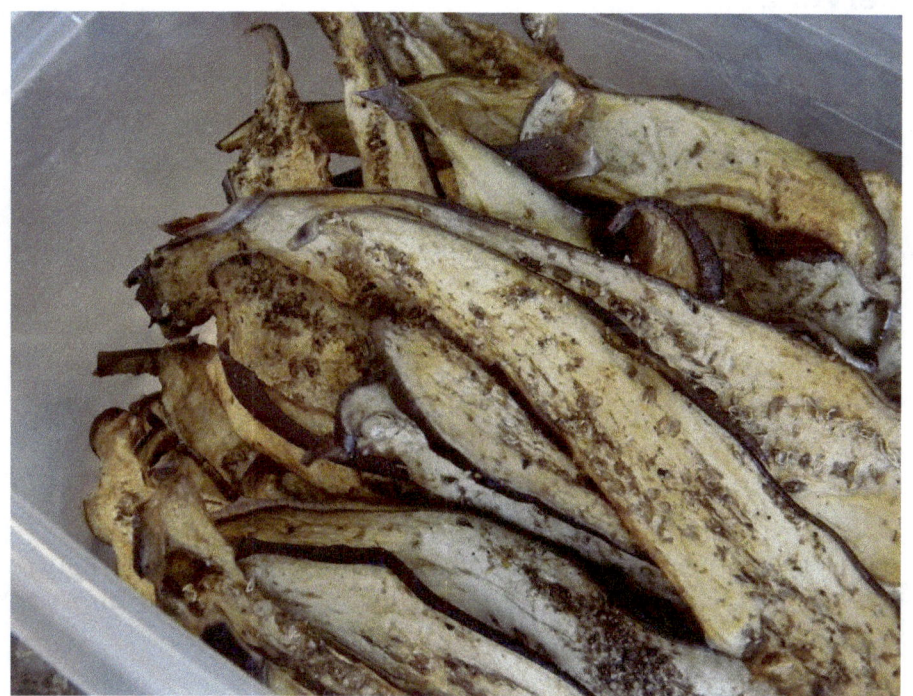

Curried Apple Chips

Preparation Time:

10 minutes

Cooking Time:

8 hours

Serve: 2

Ingredients:

1 apple, cut into

1/5-inch thick slices

1 tsp water

1 tsp cinnamon

1 tsp curry powder

Directions:

1.In a small bowl, mix together curry powder, cinnamon, and water.

2.Brush apple slices with curry powder mixture. Arrange apple slices in the air fryer basket. Select Dehydrate mode.

3.Set time to 8 hours and temperature 135 F then press START. Store in an airtight container.

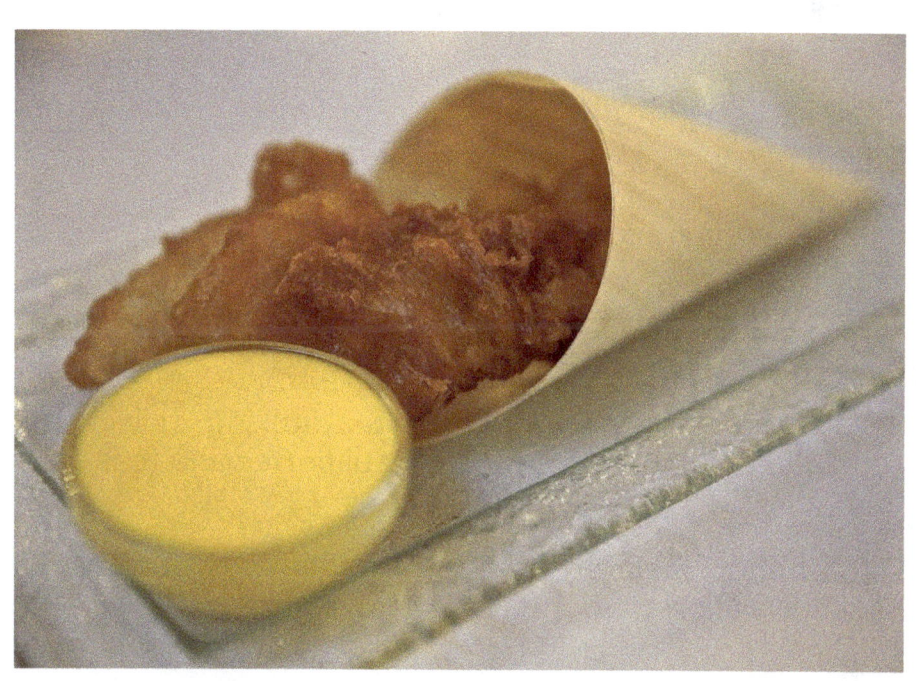

Delicious Cauliflower Popcorn

Preparation Time:

10 minutes

Cooking Time:

12 hours

Serve: 2

Ingredients:

2 cups cauliflower florets

1 tbsp nutritional yeast

1 tbsp olive oil

Pinch of cayenne pepper

Salt

Directions:

1. Add cauliflower florets into the mixing bowl. Add remaining ingredients over the cauliflower and toss well.

2. Place the cooking tray in the air fryer basket. Arrange cauliflower florets in the air fryer basket.

3. Select Dehydrate mode. Set time to 12 hours and temperature 115 F then press START. Store in an airtight container

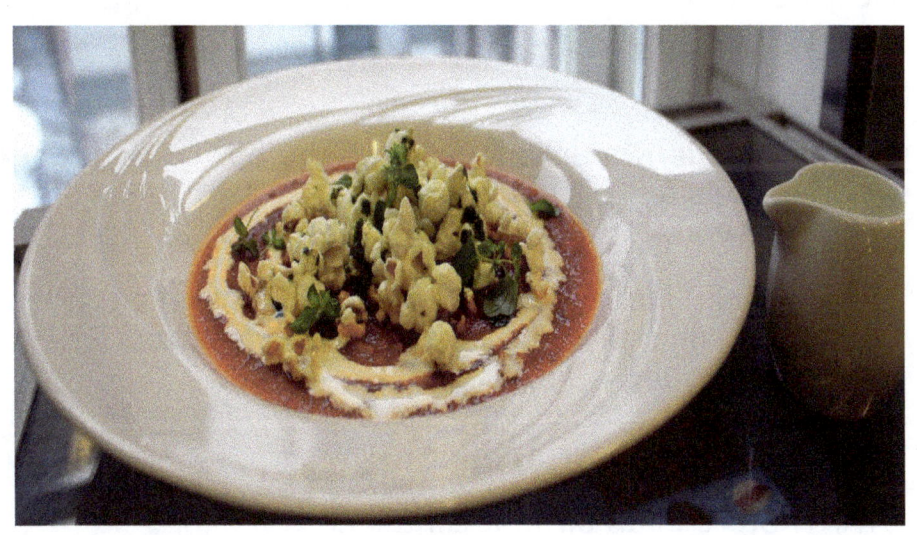

Healthy Dehydrated Almonds

Preparation Time:

10 minutes

Cooking Time:

18 hours

Serve: 4

Ingredients:

1 cup of raw almonds

2 cups of water

1 tbsp salt

Directions:

1. Add almonds, water, and salt into the bowl. Cover and soak almonds for 24 hours.

2. Drain well. Place the cooking tray in the air fryer basket. Arrange almonds in the air fryer basket. Select Dehydrate mode.

3. Set time to 18 hours and temperature 115 F then press START. Store in an airtight container.

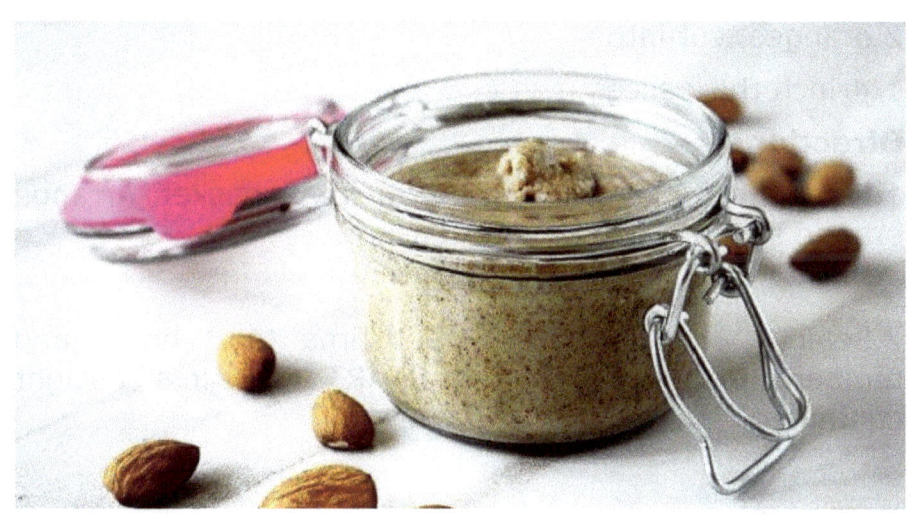

Orange Slices

Preparation Time:

10 minutes

Cooking Time:

7 hours

Serve: 2

Ingredients:

2 oranges, cut into

1/4-inch thick slices

Directions:

1. Place the cooking tray in the air fryer basket. Arrange orange slices in the air fryer basket.

2. Select Dehydrate mode. Set time to 7 hours and temperature 135 F then press START. Store in an airtight container.

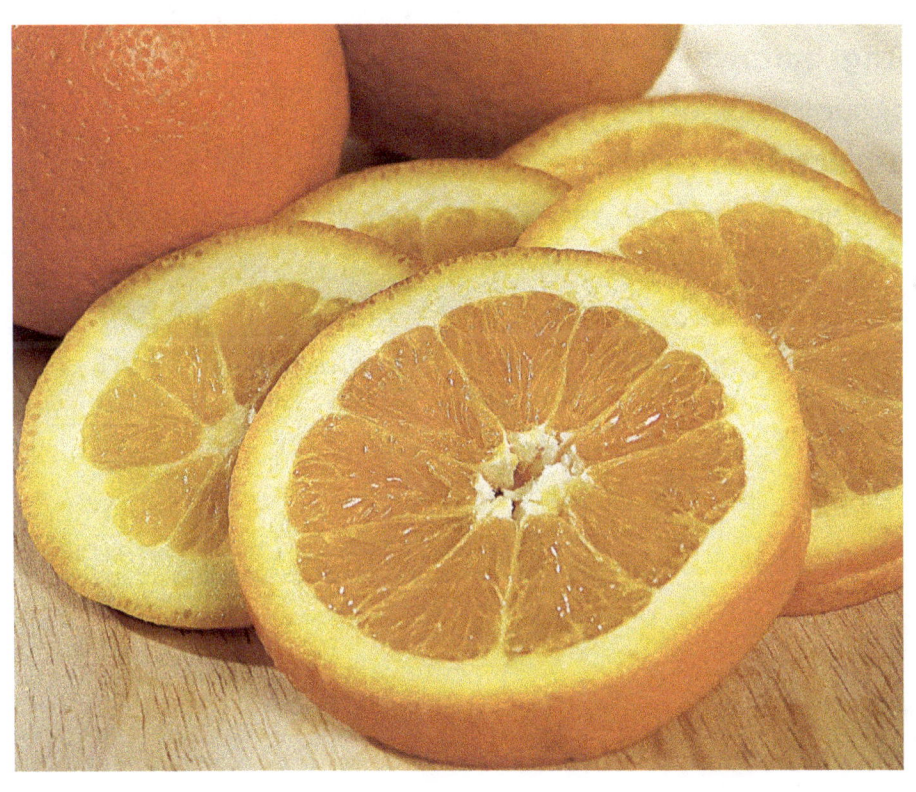

Dried Raspberries

Preparation Time:

10 minutes

Cooking Time:

8 hours

Serve: 4

Ingredients:

2 cups raspberries, cut in half

Directions:

1. Place the cooking tray in the air fryer basket. Arrange raspberries in the air fryer basket.

2. Select Dehydrate mode. Set time to 8 hours and temperature 135 F then press START. Store in an airtight container.

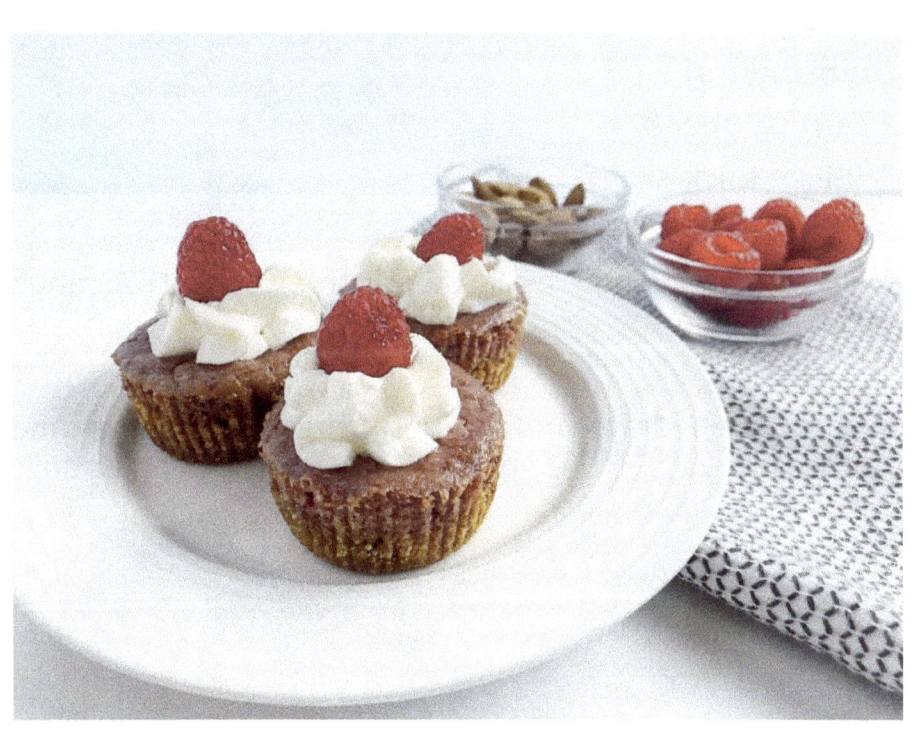

Dehydrated Carrot Slices

Preparation Time:

10 minutes

Cooking Time:

6 hours

Serve: 4

Ingredients:

2 carrots, peel &

1/8-inch thick slices

Directions:

1.Place the cooking tray in the air fryer basket. Arrange carrot slices in the air fryer basket.

2.Select Dehydrate mode. Set time to 6 hours and temperature 125 F then press START. Store in an airtight container.

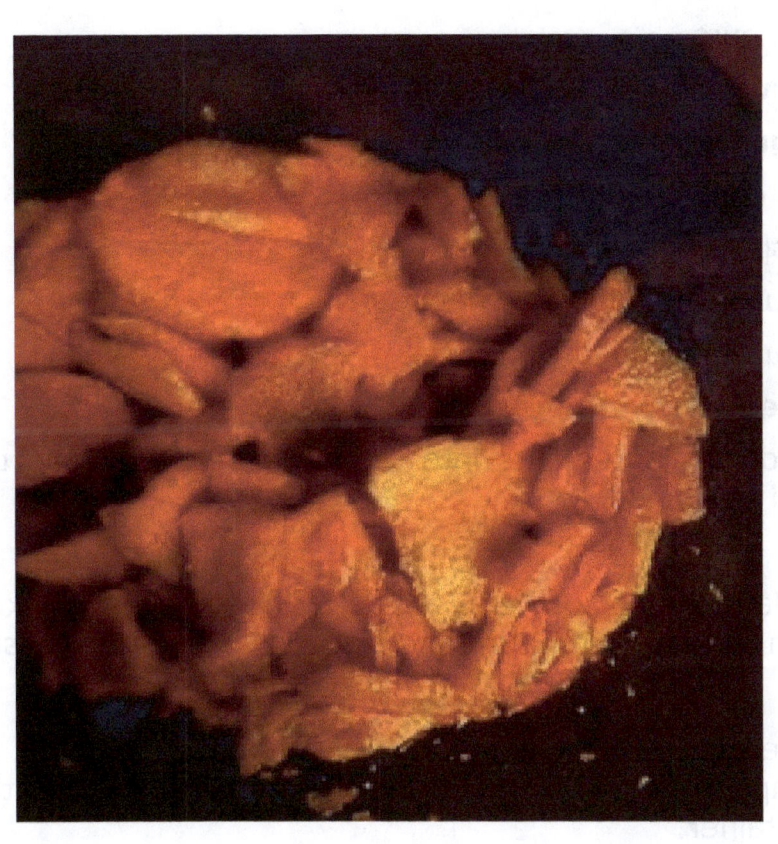

Coconut Peanut Butter Balls

Preparation Time:

10 minutes

Cooking Time:

12 hours

Serve: 5

Ingredients:

2/3 cups peanut butter

1 tsp vanilla

2 cups dried apples, chopped

2 cups shredded coconut

Directions:

1. Add all ingredients into the large bowl and mix until well combined.

2. Place the cooking tray in the air fryer basket. Make 1-inch balls from mixture and place in the air fryer basket.

3. Select Dehydrate mode. Set time to 12 hours and temperature 135 F then press START. Store in an airtight container.

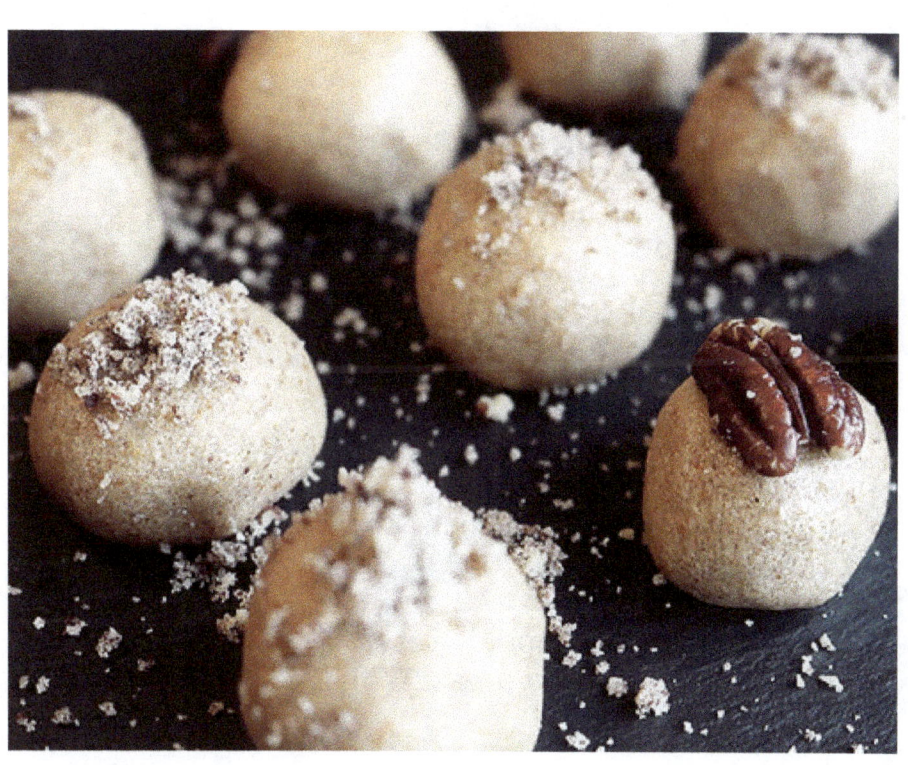

Spicy Rosemary Almonds

Preparation Time:

10 minutes

Cooking Time:

24 hours

Serve: 6

Ingredients:

2 cups almonds, soak in water for overnight

1 tbsp fresh rosemary, chopped

1 tsp chili powder

1 tbsp olive oil

3/4 tsp kosher salt

Directions:

1. Add all ingredients into the mixing bowl and toss well. Place the cooking tray in the air fryer basket. Spread almonds in the air fryer basket.

2. Select Dehydrate mode. Set time to 24 hours and temperature 125 F then press START. Store in an airtight container

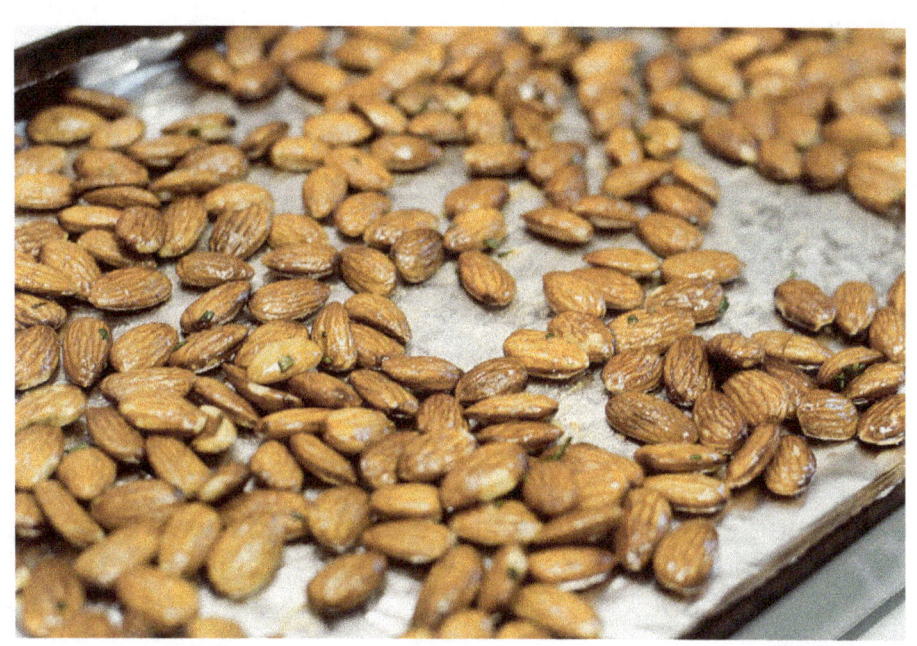

Lemon Avocado Chips

Preparation Time:

10 minutes

Cooking Time:

10 hours

Serve: 4

Ingredients:

4 avocados, halved and pitted

1/4 tsp cayenne pepper

1/2 lemon juice

1/4 tsp sea salt

Directions:

1.Cut avocado into the slices. Drizzle lemon juice over avocado slices. Place the cooking tray in the air fryer basket.

2.Arrange avocado slices in the air fryer basket. Sprinkle cayenne pepper and salt over avocado slices. Select Dehydrate mode.

3.Set time to 10 hours and temperature 160 F then press START. Store in an airtight container.

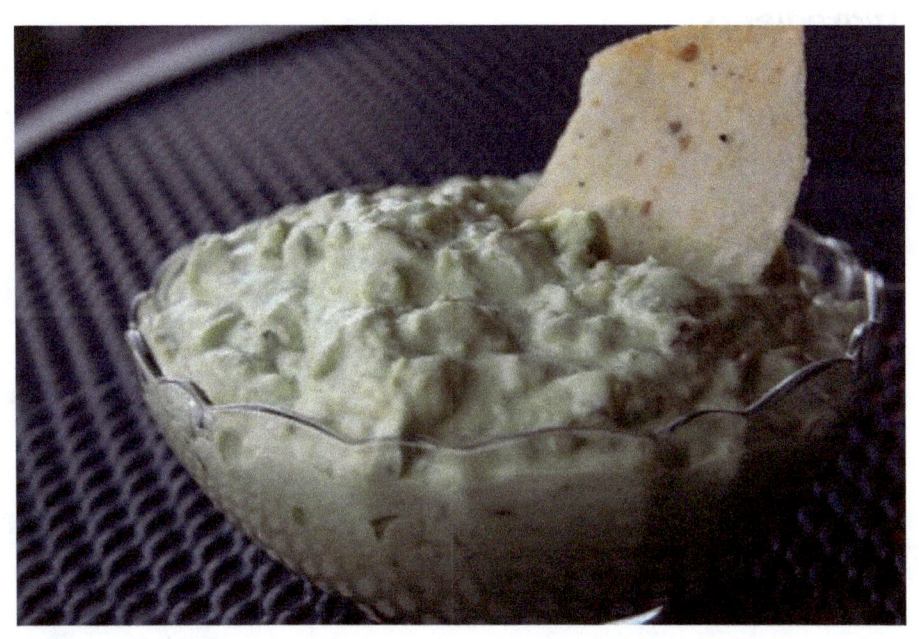

Smokey Tofu Jerky

Preparation Time:

10 minutes

Cooking Time:

4 hours

Serve: 4

Ingredients:

1 block tofu, pressed & Cut in half then cut into the slices
2 tbsp Worcestershire sauce

2 tbsp sriracha

4 drops liquid smoke

Directions:

1. In a bowl, mix together liquid smoke, sriracha, and Worcestershire sauce.

2. Add tofu slices in a bowl and mix until well coated. Cover bowl and place in the refrigerator overnight. Place the cooking tray in the air fryer basket.

3. Arrange marinated tofu slices in the air fryer basket. Select Dehydrate mode. Set time to 4 hours and temperature 145 F then press START. Store in an airtight container.

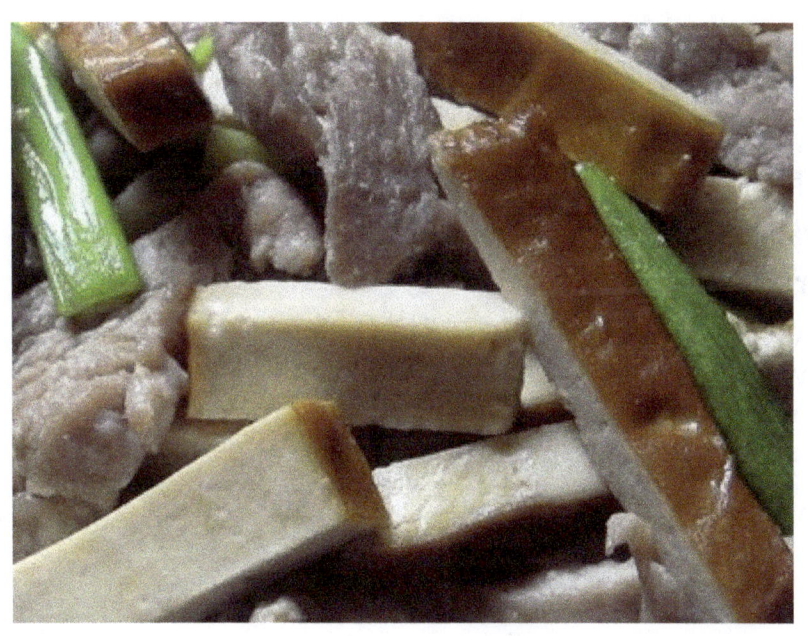

Parmesan Zucchini Chips

Preparation Time:

10 minutes

Cooking Time:

10 hours

Serve: 2

Ingredients:

1 zucchini, sliced thinly

2 tbsp parmesan cheese, grated

1 tsp vinegar

1/8 tsp garlic powder Salt

Directions:

1. Add zucchini slices, parmesan cheese, vinegar, garlic powder, and salt into the bowl and toss well. Place the cooking tray in the air fryer basket.

2. Arrange zucchini slices in the air fryer basket. Select Dehydrate mode.

3. Set time to 10 hours and temperature 135 F then press START. Store in an airtight container

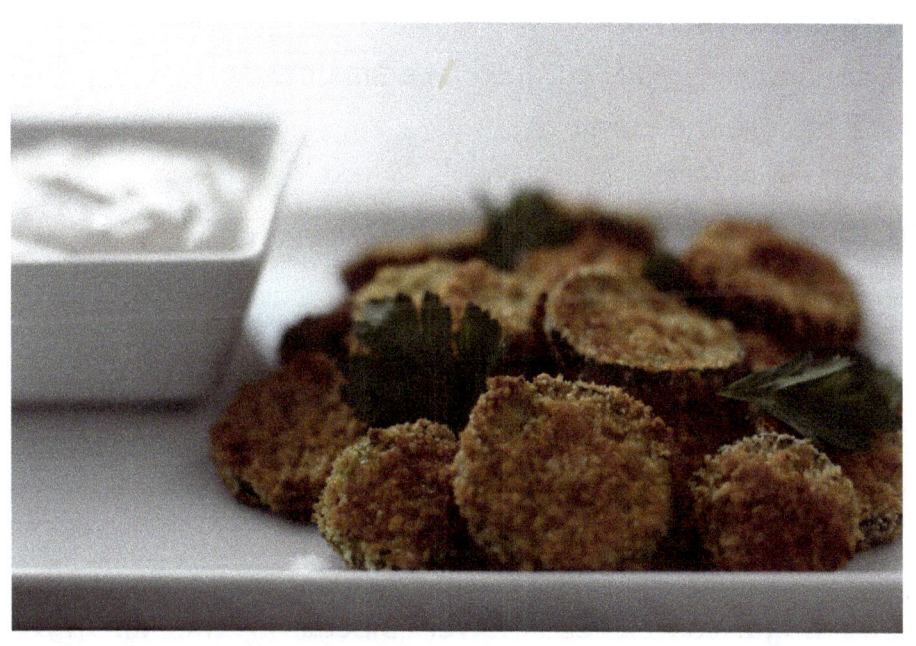

Spicy Cauliflower Popcorn

Preparation Time:

10 minutes

Cooking Time:

12 hours

Serve: 4

Ingredients:

1 cauliflower head, cut into bite-size pieces

1/2 tsp ground cumin

1 tsp cayenne

1 tbsp paprika

1/4 cup hot sauce

3 tbsp coconut oil

Directions:

1. Add cauliflower pieces into the large mixing bowl. Add remaining ingredients and toss until well coated. Place the cooking tray in the air fryer basket.

2. Arrange coated cauliflower pieces in the air fryer basket. Select Dehydrate mode. Set time to 12 hours and temperature 130 F then press START. Store in an airtight container

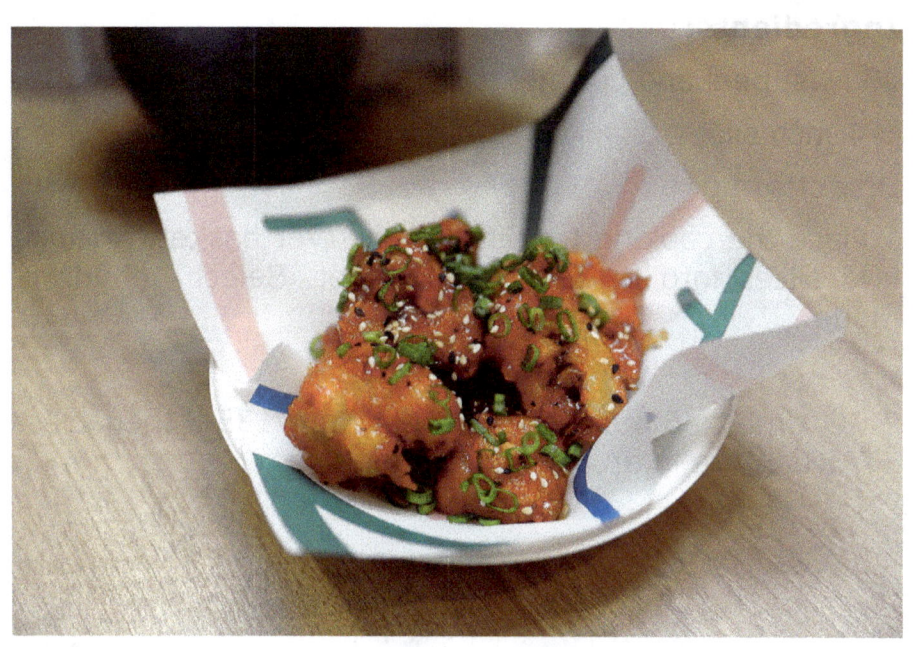

Easy Kiwi Chips

Preparation Time:

10 minutes

Cooking Time:

6 hours

Serve: 4

Ingredients:

4 kiwis, peel and cut into

1/4-inch slices

Directions:

1.Place the cooking tray in the air fryer basket. Arrange kiwi slices into the air fryer basket. Select Dehydrate mode.

2.Set time to 6 hours and temperature 135 F then press START. Store in an airtight container.

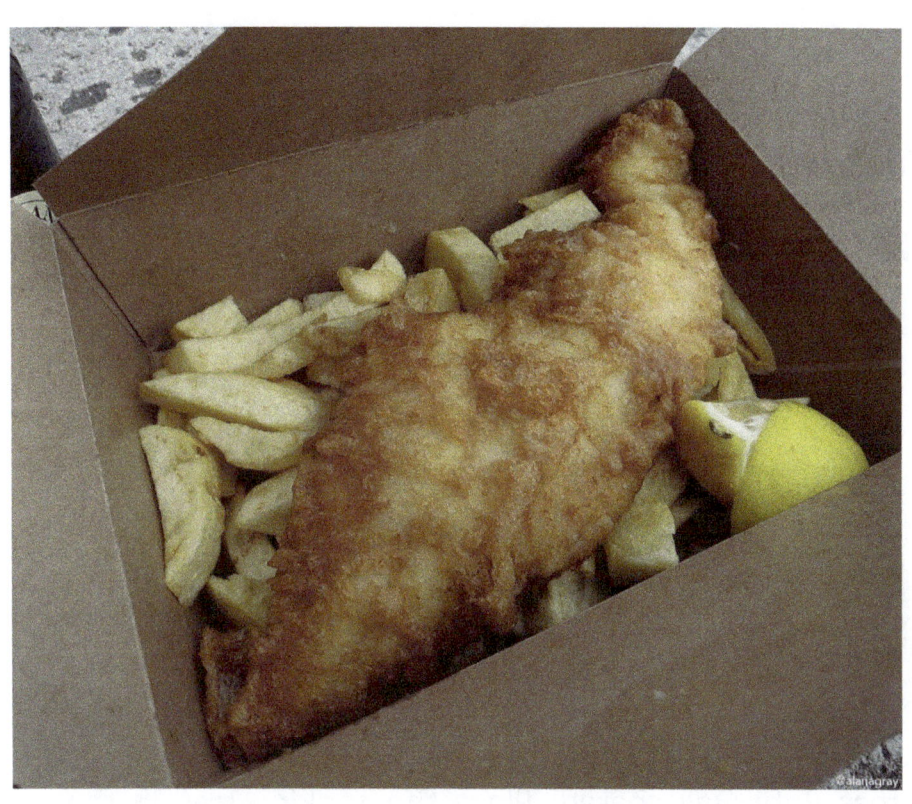

Crunchy Broccoli Chips

Preparation Time:

10 minutes

Cooking Time:

12 hours

Serve: 4

Ingredients:

1 lb broccoli florets

1 tsp onion powder

1 garlic clove

1/2 cup vegetable broth

1/4 cup hemp seeds

2 tbsp nutritional yeast

2 tbsp low-sodium tamari sauce

Directions:

1.Add hemp seeds, tamari sauce, nutritional yeast, broth, garlic, and onion powder into the blender and blend until smooth.

2.Pour sauce over broccoli florets in a mixing bowl and toss until well coated. Place the cooking tray in the air fryer basket. Place piece of parchment paper into the air fryer basket.

3.Arrange broccoli florets in the air fryer basket. Select Dehydrate mode. Set time to 10-12 hours and temperature 115 F then press START. Store in an airtight container.

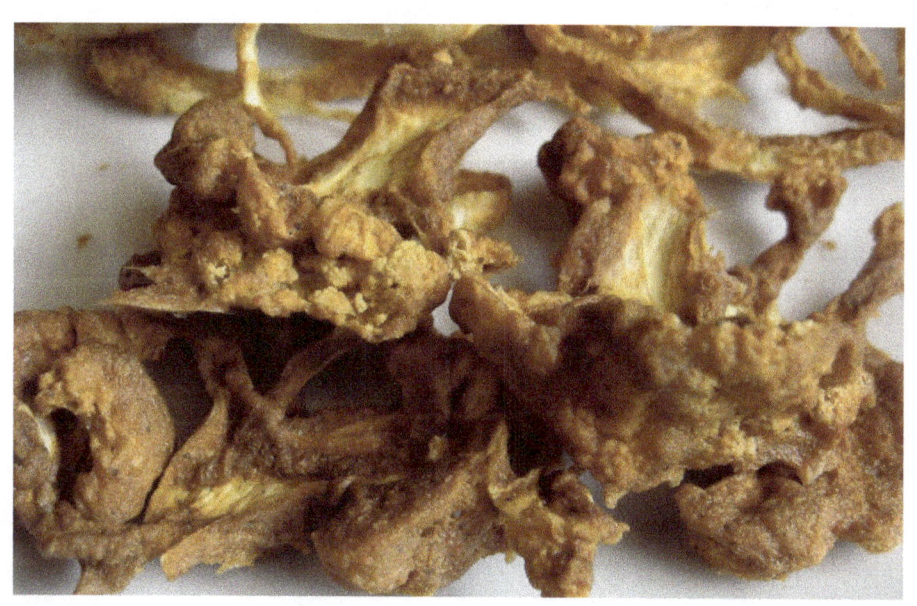

Cabbage Chips

Preparation Time:

10 minutes

Cooking Time:

12 hours

Serve: 4

Ingredients:

1/2 lb napa cabbage, cut stem, wash & dry leaves

1/2 tsp ground pepper

1 tbsp olive oil

1/2 tsp salt

Directions:

1. Cut cabbage leaves in a triangle shape. Toss cabbage leaves with olive oil, pepper, and salt. Place the cooking tray in the air fryer basket.

2. Arrange cabbage leaves in the air fryer basket. Select Dehydrate mode. Set time to 12 hours and temperature 135 F then press START.

3. Store in an airtight container.

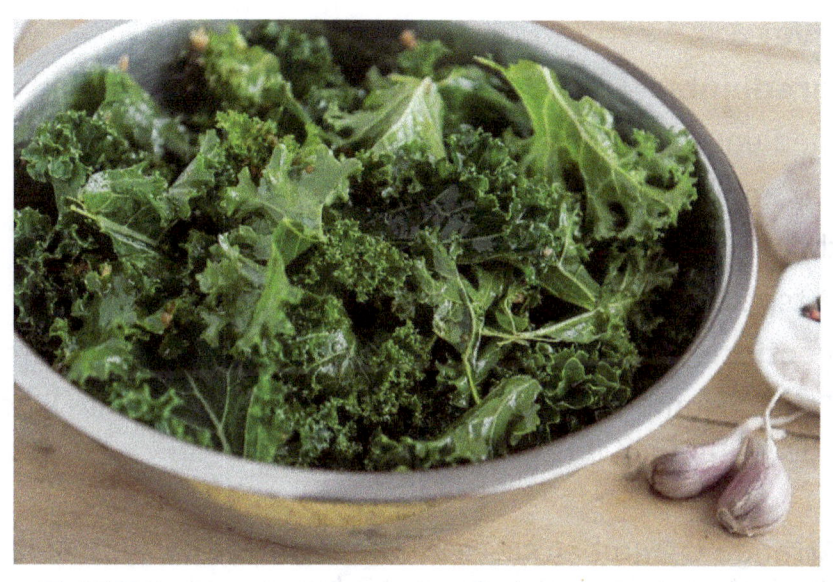

Healthy Cucumber Chips

Preparation Time:

10 minutes

Cooking Time:

12 hours

Serve: 6

Ingredients:

2 medium cucumbers, thinly sliced

2 tsp apple cider vinegar

1 tbsp olive oil

1/2 tsp sea salt

Directions:

1. Toss cucumber slices with vinegar, oil, and salt. Place the cooking tray in the air fryer basket.

2. Arrange cucumber slices in the air fryer basket. Select Dehydrate mode. Set time to 12 hours and temperature 125 F then press START. Store in an airtight container.

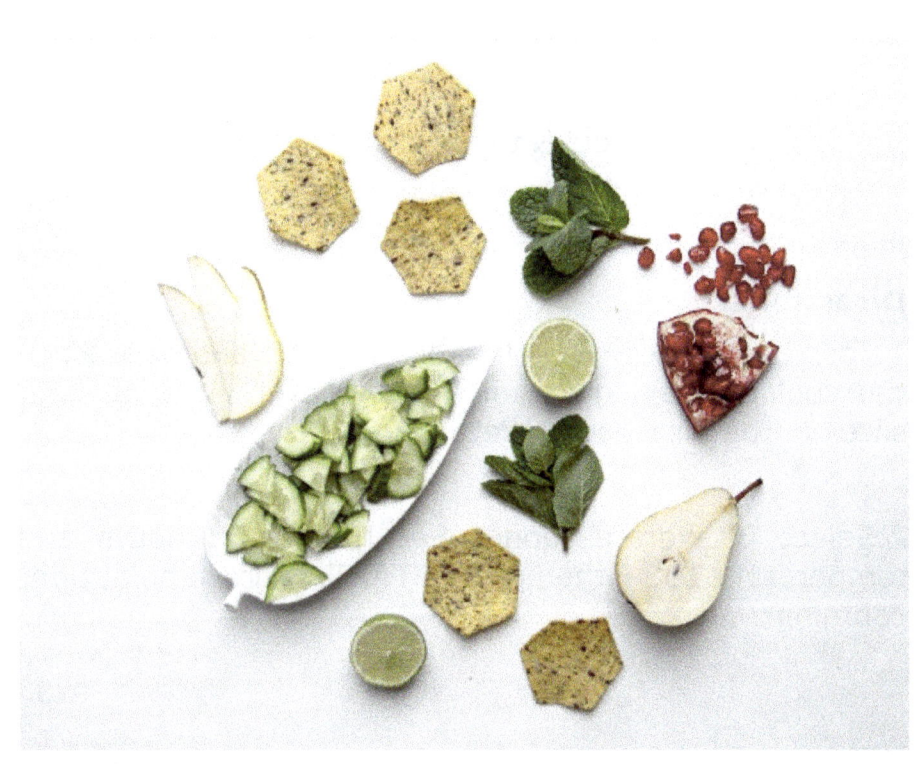

Beet Chips

Preparation Time:

10 minutes

Cooking Time:

8 hours

Serve: 4

Ingredients:

3 medium beets, peel & thinly sliced

1 tsp olive oil

Pepper Salt

Directions:

1. Toss beet slices with olive oil, pepper, and salt. Place the cooking tray in the air fryer basket. Arrange beet slices in the air fryer basket.

2. Select Dehydrate mode. Set time to 8 hours and temperature 130 F then press START. Store in an airtight container.

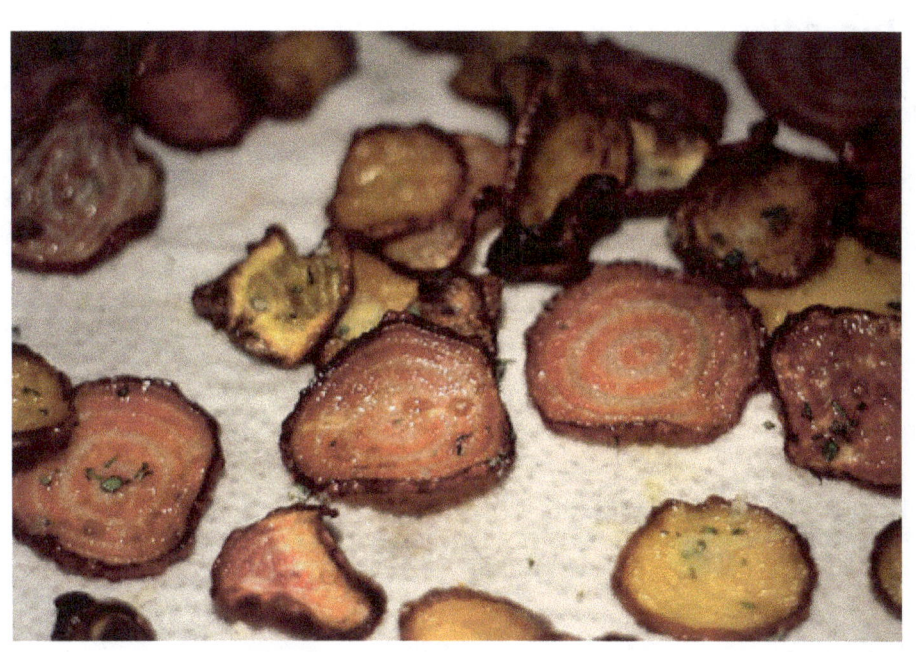

Tasty Tomato Chips

Preparation Time:

10 minutes

Cooking Time:

8 hours

Serve: 4

Ingredients:

3 large tomatoes, cut into 1.5 mm slices

For sauce:

1/2 cup cashews, soaked for 2 hours and drain

1/2 tsp red pepper flakes

1 tsp paprika

1 tsp dried oregano

2 tbsp nutritional yeast

2 tbsp lemon juice

2 cups red bell pepper, chopped

1/4 cup water

1/4 tsp salt

Directions:

1. Add all sauce ingredients into the blender and blend until smooth. Place the cooking tray in the air fryer basket.

2. Place piece of parchment paper into the air fryer basket. Dredge tomato slices into the sauce.

3.Drip off excess sauce and arrange tomato slices onto the parchment paper in the air fryer basket. Select Dehydrate mode.

4.Set time to 8 hours and temperature 115 F then press START. Store in an airtight container.

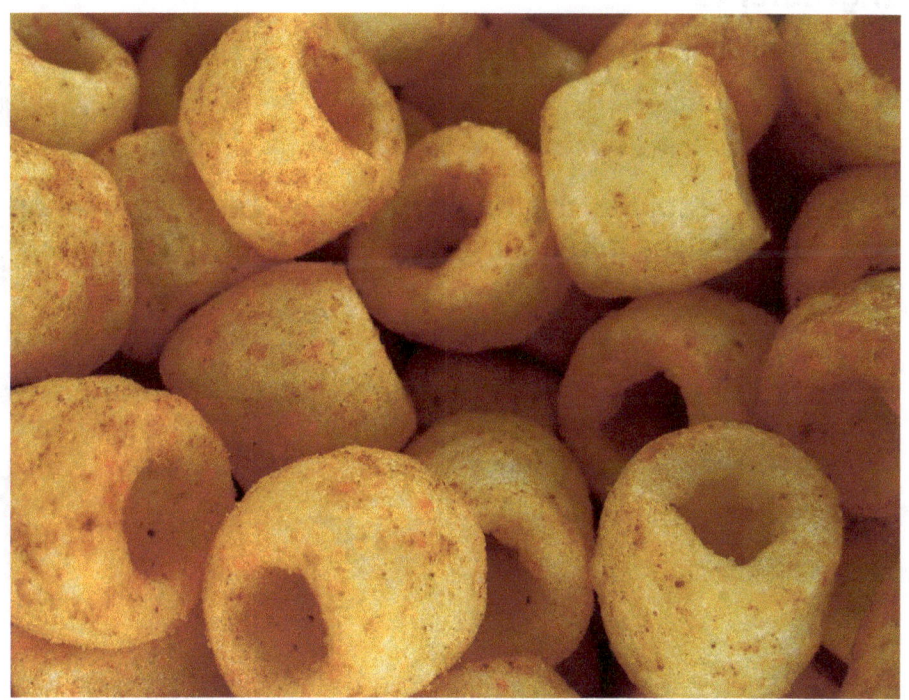

Strawberry Chips

Preparation Time:

10 minutes

Cooking Time:

3 hours

Serve: 4

Ingredients:

8 fresh strawberries, cut into 1/8-inch slices

Directions:

1. Place the cooking tray in the air fryer basket. Arrange strawberry slices in the air fryer basket. Select Dehydrate mode.

2. Set time to 3 hours and temperature 125 F then press START. Store in an airtight container.

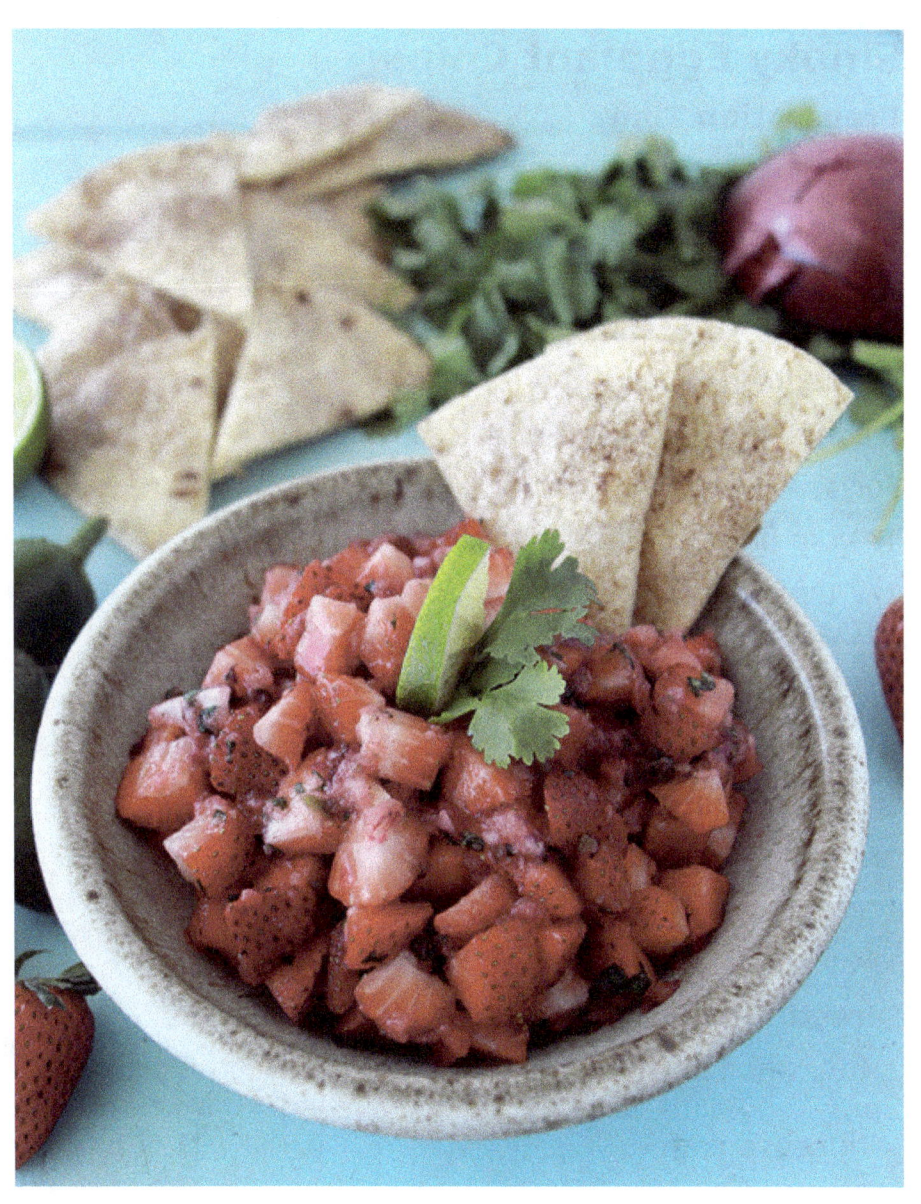

Smoky Eggplant Chips

Preparation Time:

10 minutes

Cooking Time:

10 hours

Serve: 4

Ingredients:

2 eggplants, cut into thin slices

For seasoning:

1/4 tsp dried ground sage

1/2 tsp onion powder

1/2 tsp pepper

1/2 tsp turmeric

1/2 tsp dried thyme

1 tsp dried oregano

1/2 tbsp garlic powder

1/2 tbsp smoked paprika

1/4 tsp sea salt

Directions:

1. In a small bowl, mix together all seasoning ingredients. Spray eggplant slices with cooking spray and sprinkle with seasoning.

2. Place the cooking tray in the air fryer basket. Arrange eggplant slices in the air fryer basket. Select Dehydrate mode.

3.Set time to 10 hours and temperature 115 F then press START. Store in an airtight container.

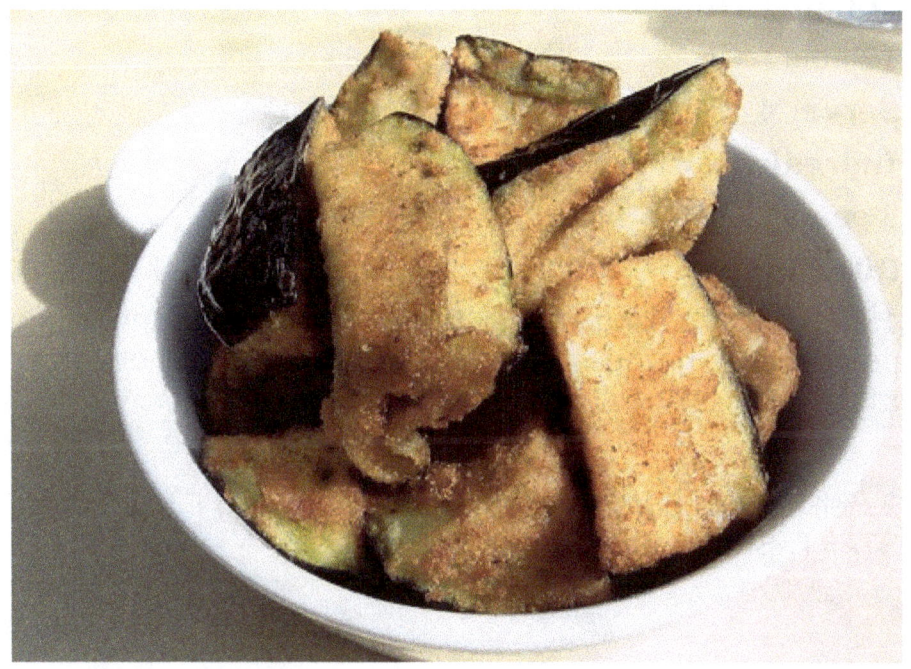

Pear Chips

Preparation Time:

10 minutes

Cooking Time:

10 hours

Serve: 4

Ingredients:

3 pears, cut into slices

Directions:

1. Place the cooking tray in the air fryer basket. Arrange pear slices in the air fryer basket. Select Dehydrate mode.

2. Set time to 8 hours and temperature 130 F then press START. Store in an airtight container

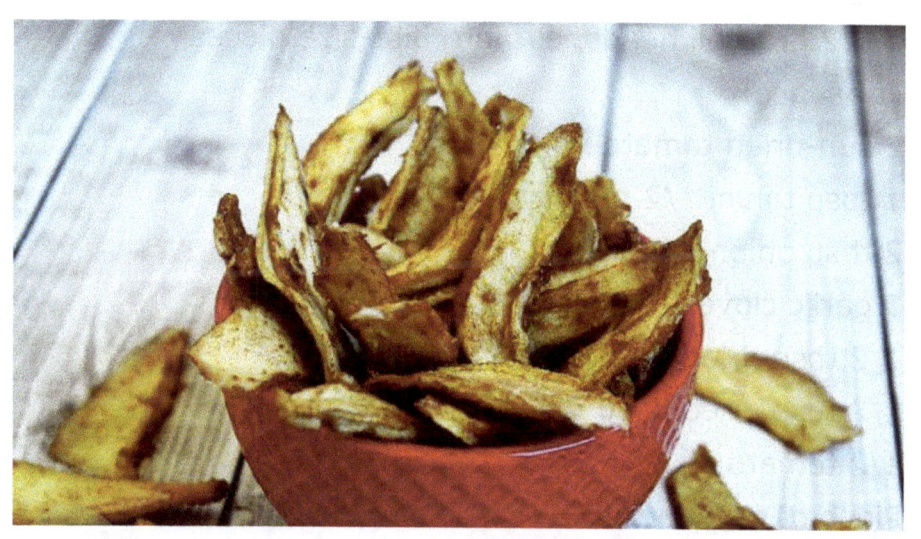

Broccoli Bites

Preparation Time:

10 minutes

Cooking Time:

18 hours

Serve: 3

Ingredients:

1 1/2 broccoli heads, cut into bite-size pieces

For sauce:

2 sun-dried tomatoes

1 tbsp tahini 1/2 tbsp paprika

2 tbsp onion, chopped

1 garlic clove

1/2 tbsp dried oregano

1/2 tbsp dried basil

1/2 tomato

Pinch of cayenne

Directions:

1. Add all sauce ingredients into the blender and blend until smooth.

2. Add broccoli pieces into the mixing bowl. Pour sauce over broccoli and toss until well coated. Place the cooking tray in the air fryer basket.

3. Arrange broccoli in the air fryer basket. Select Dehydrate mode. Set time to 18 hours and temperature 110 F then press START. Store in an airtight container.

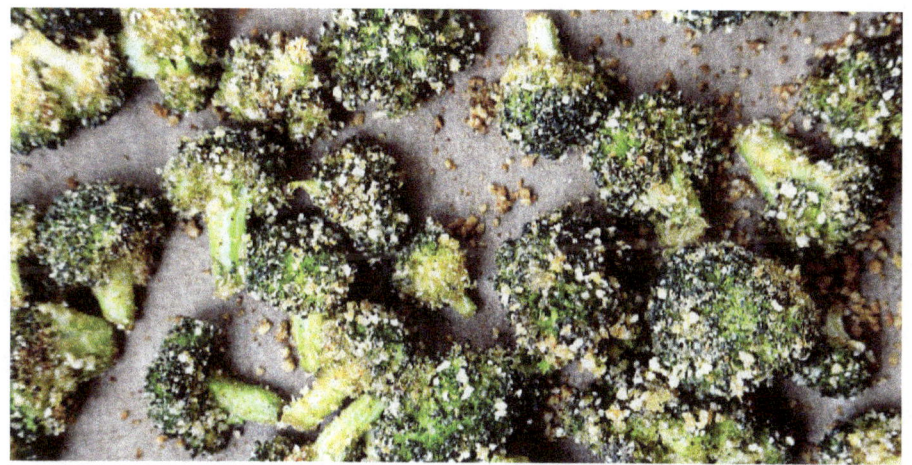

Chili Lime Cauliflower Popcorn

Preparation Time:

10 minutes

Cooking Time:

12 hours

Serve: 4

Ingredients:

1 large cauliflower head, cut into florets

1 tbsp chili powder

1 tbsp olive oil

1 lime juice

1 tsp sea salt

Directions:

1. Add cauliflower florets into the mixing bowl. Add remaining ingredients and toss well. Place the cooking tray in the air fryer basket.

2. Arrange cauliflower florets in the air fryer basket. Select Dehydrate mode. Set time to 12 hours and temperature 135 F then press START. Store in an airtight container.

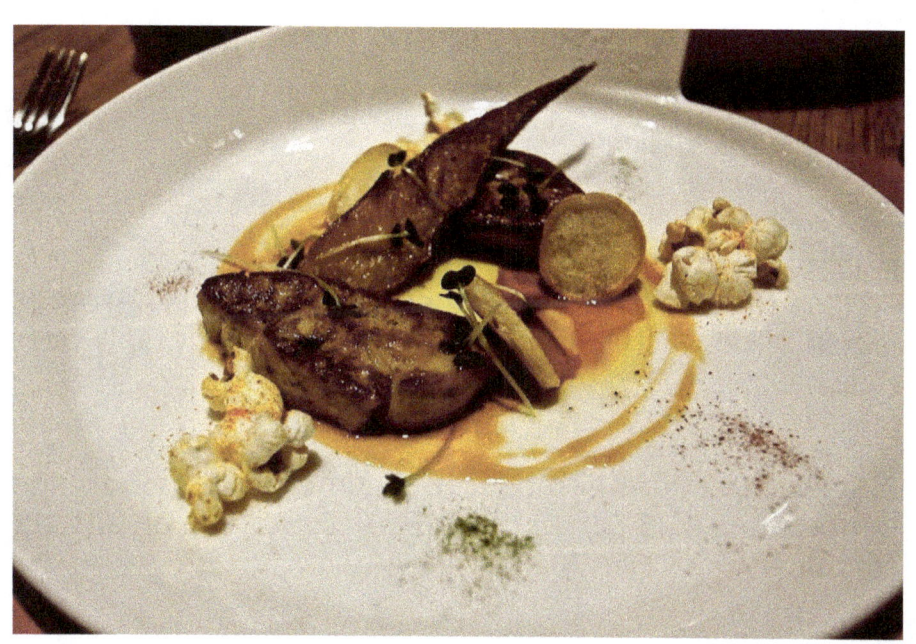

Radish Chips

Preparation Time:

10 minutes

Cooking Time:

5 hours

Serve: 4

Ingredients:

3 radishes, cut into

1/8-inch thick slices

Salt

Directions:

1. Place the cooking tray in the air fryer basket. Arrange radish slices in the air fryer basket. Sprinkle salt over radish slices.

2. Select Dehydrate mode. Set time to 5 hours and temperature 125 F then press START. Store in an airtight container

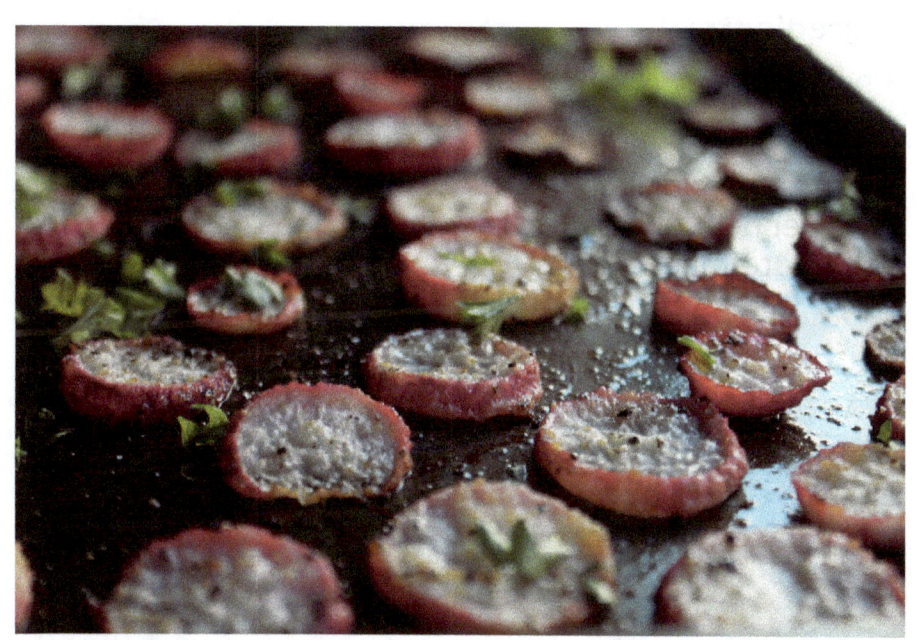

Dehydrated Bell Peppers

Preparation Time:

10 minutes

Cooking Time:

8 hours

Serve: 3

Ingredients:

3 bell peppers, remove seeds & cut into slices

Directions:

1. Place the cooking tray in the air fryer basket. Arrange bell pepper slices in the air fryer basket. Select Dehydrate mode.

2. Set time to 8 hours and temperature 125 F then press START. Store in an airtight container.

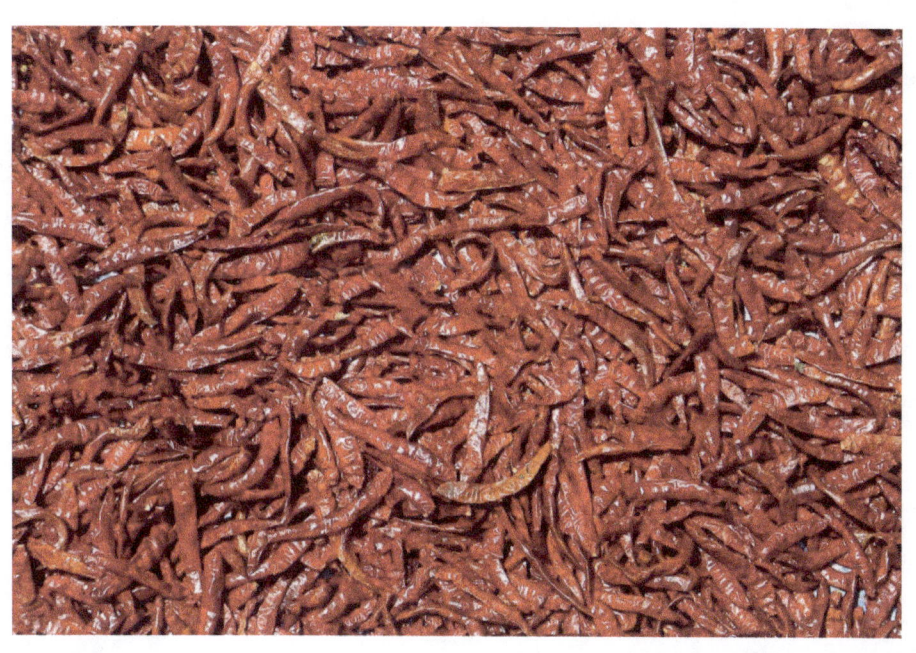

Brussels Sprout Chips

Preparation Time:

10 minutes

Cooking Time:

10 hours

Serve: 4

Ingredients:

1 lb Brussel sprouts, cut the stem and separate leaves

1 tsp soy sauce

2 tbsp sriracha

Pinch of salt

Directions:

1. In a mixing bowl, toss Brussel sprouts with soy sauce, sriracha, and salt. Place the cooking tray in the air fryer basket.

2. Arrange Brussels sprouts in the air fryer basket. Select Dehydrate mode. Set time to 10 hours and temperature 115 F then press START. Store in airtight container.

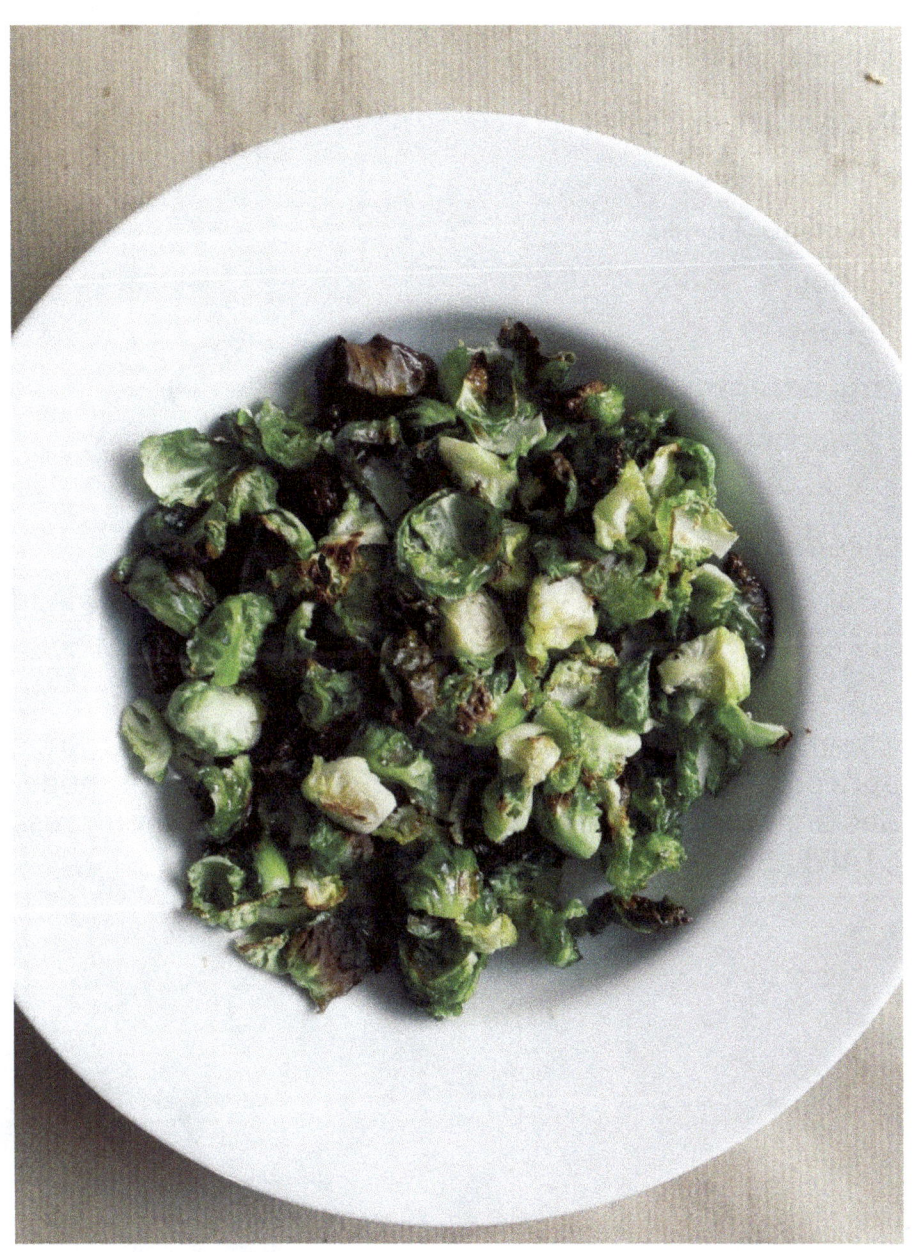

Dried Apricots

Preparation Time:

10 minutes

Cooking Time:

20 hours

Serve: 12

Ingredients:

12 apricots, cut in half & remove pits

4 cups of water 1 cup lemon juice

Directions:

1. In a large bowl, add water and lemon juice. Add apricots.

2. Remove apricots from water and pat dry. Arrange apricots in the air fryer basket. Select Dehydrate mode. Set time to 20 hours and temperature 135 F then press START. Store in an airtight container.

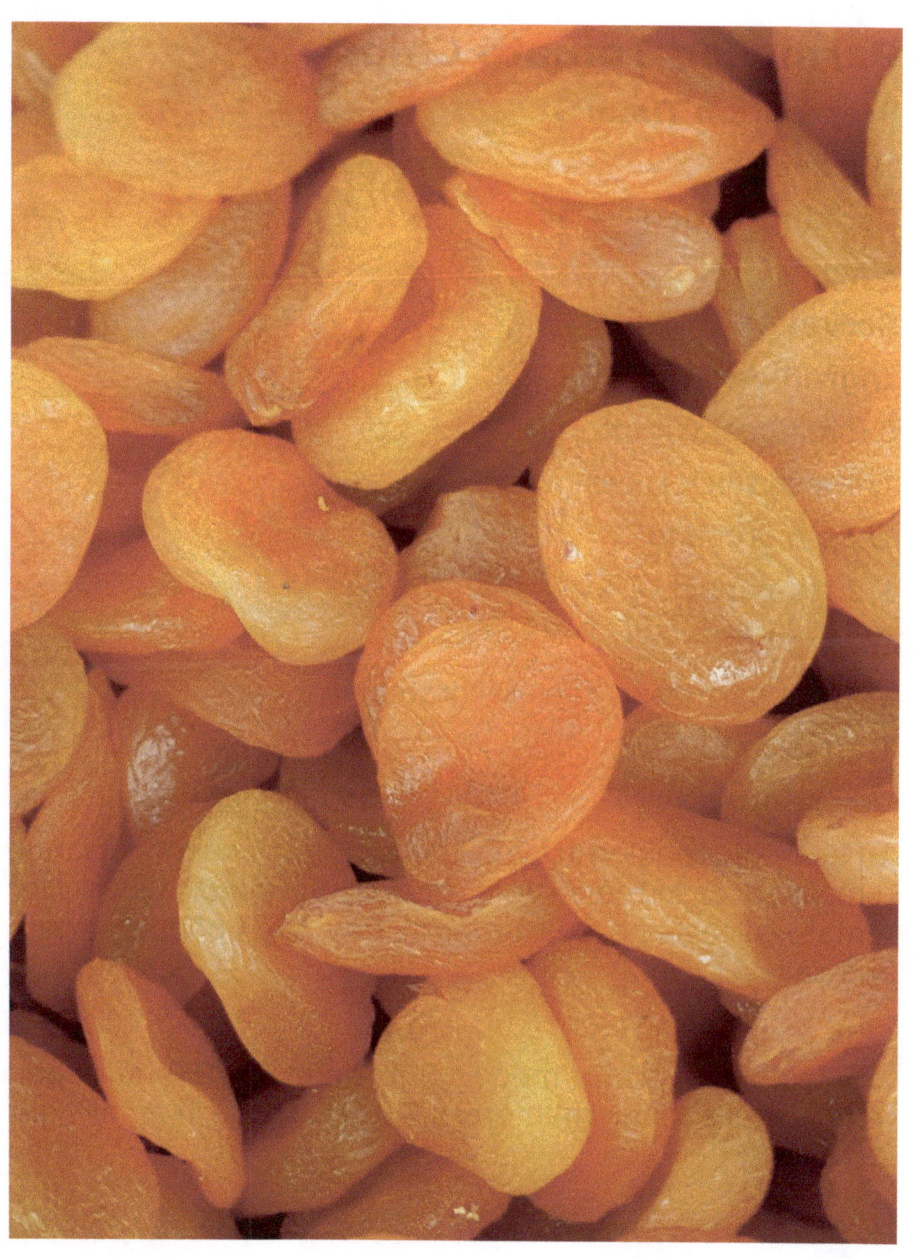

Parmesan Tomato Chips

Preparation Time:

10 minutes

Cooking Time:

8 hours

Serve: 6

Ingredients:

8 tomatoes, cut into 1/4-inch thick slices

1/2 tsp oregano

1/2 tsp pepper

1/2 tsp basil

1/4 cup parmesan cheese, grated

1/2 tsp salt

Directions:

1.Place the cooking tray in the air fryer basket. Arrange tomato slices in the air fryer basket. Sprinkle cheese over tomato slices and season with oregano, pepper, basil, and salt.

2.Select Dehydrate mode. Set time to 8 hours and temperature 155 F then press START. Store in an airtight container.

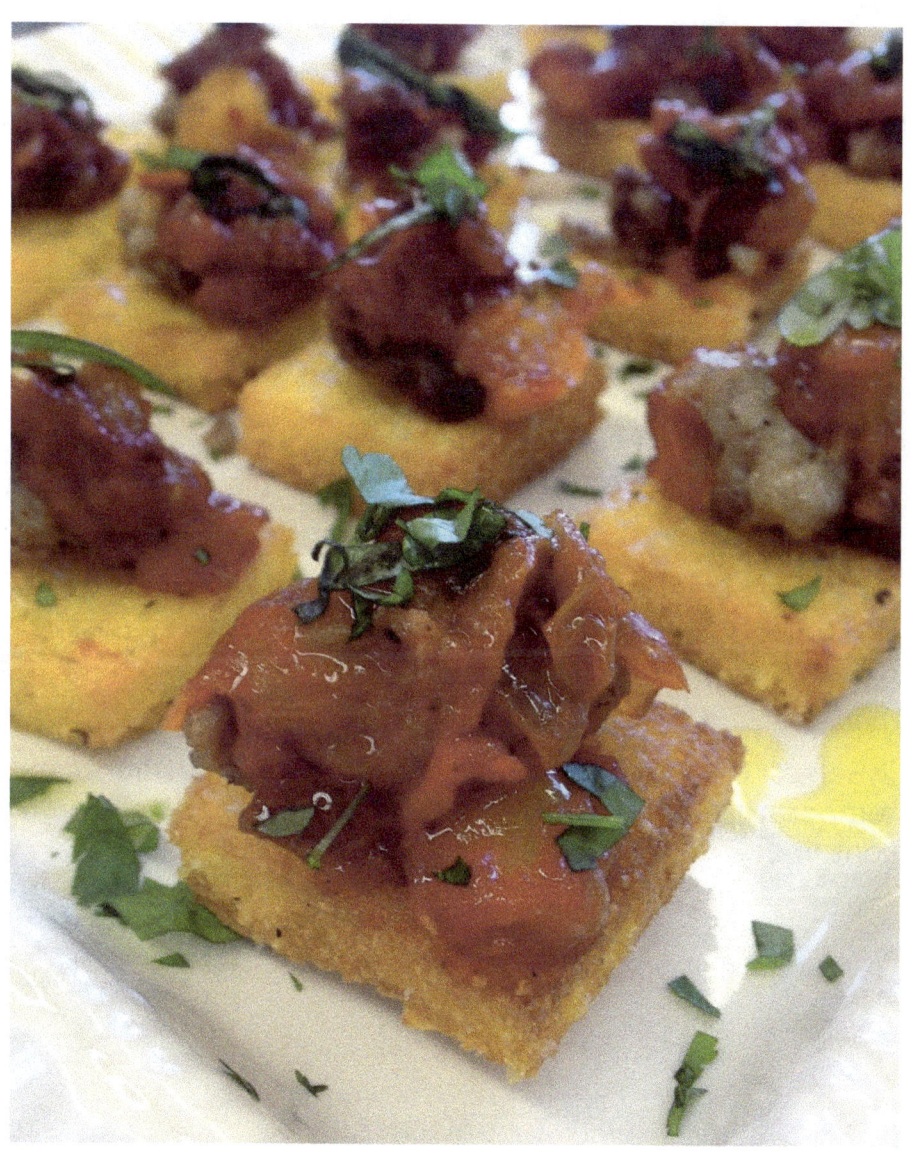

Dehydrated Raspberries

Preparation Time:

10 minutes

Cooking Time:

18 hours

Serve: 4

Ingredients:

4 cups raspberries, wash and dry

1/4 cup fresh lemon juice

Directions:

1. Add raspberries and lemon juice in a bowl and mix well. Place the cooking tray in the air fryer basket. Arrange raspberries in the air fryer basket.

2. Select Dehydrate mode. Set time to 18 hours and temperature 135 F then press START. Store in an airtight container.

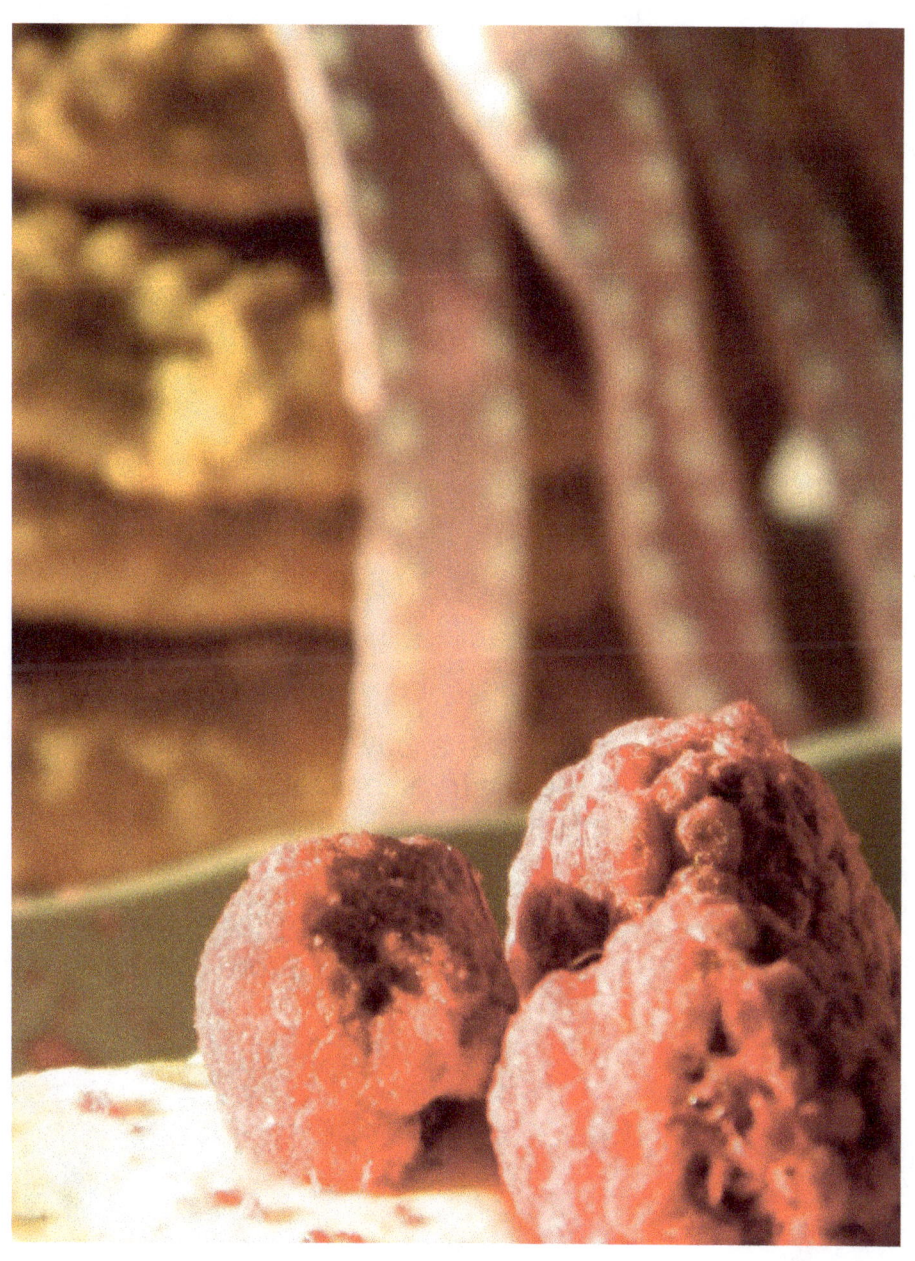

Squash Chips

Preparation Time:

10 minutes

Cooking Time:

12 hours

Serve: 8

Ingredients:

1 yellow squash, cut into

1/8-inch thick slices

2 tsp olive oil

2 tbsp vinegar

Salt

Directions:

1. Add all ingredients into the bowl and toss well. Place the cooking tray in the air fryer basket. Arrange squash slices in the air fryer basket.

2. Select Dehydrate mode. Set time to 12 hours and temperature 115 F then press START. Store in an airtight container.

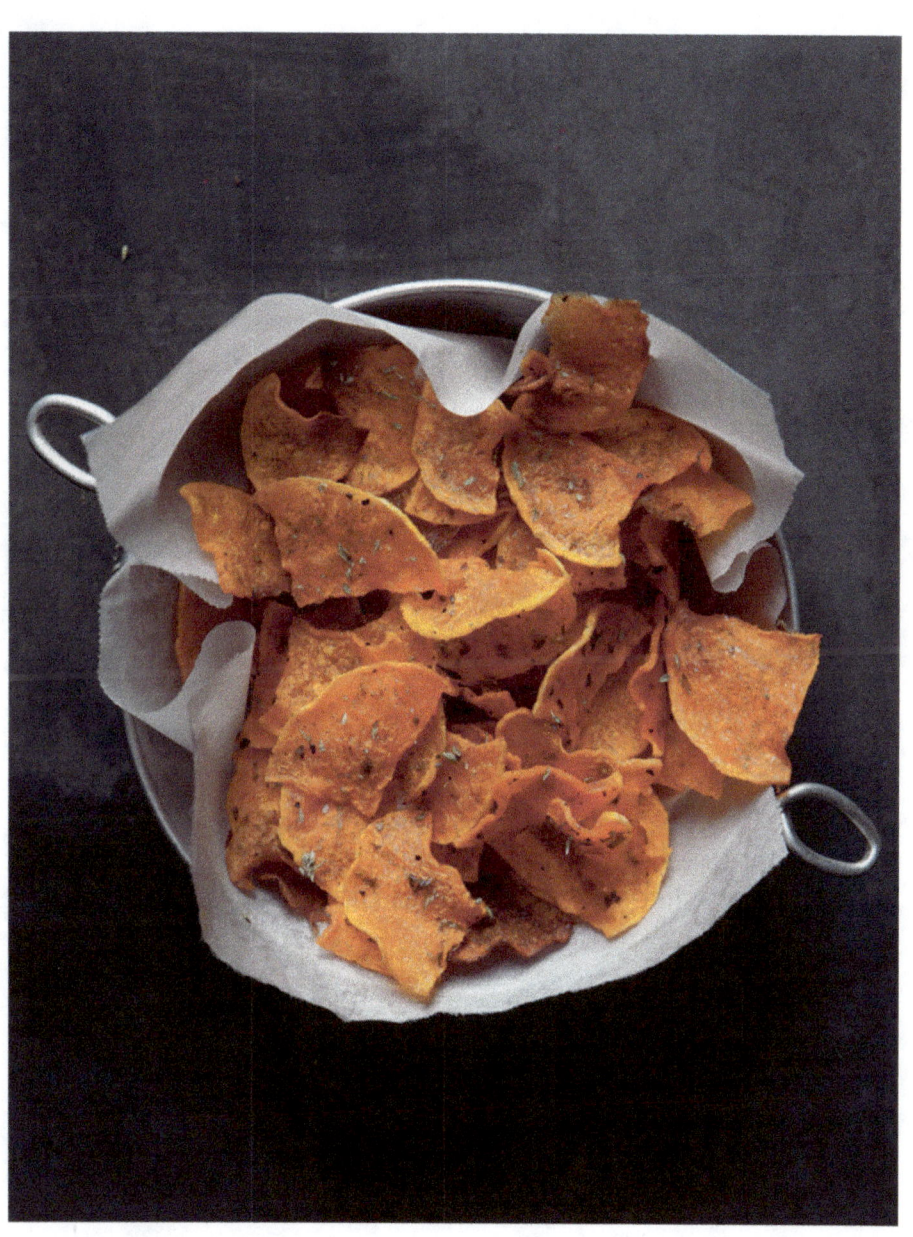

Lemon Chicken Jerky

Preparation Time:

10 minutes

Cooking Time:

7 hours

Serve: 4

Ingredients:

1 1/2 lb chicken tenders, boneless, skinless and cut into 1/4-inch slices

1/4 tsp ground ginger

1/4 tsp black pepper

1/2 tsp garlic powder

1 tsp lemon juice

1/2 cup soy sauce

Directions:

1. Mix all ingredients except chicken into the zip-lock bag. Add chicken slices, seal bag and place in the refrigerator for 30 minutes.

2. Place the cooking tray in the air fryer basket. Arrange marinated chicken slices in the air fryer basket. Select Dehydrate mode. Set time to 7 hours and temperature 145 F then press START. Store in an airtight container.

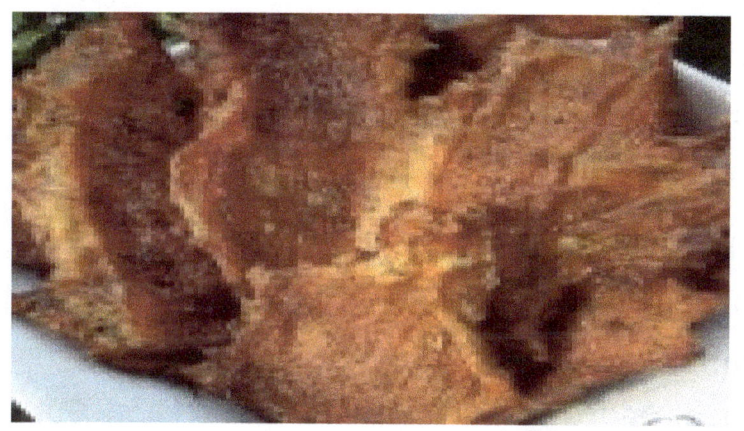

Classic Crème Brûlée

Cook Time:

30 minutes

Servings: 4

Ingredients:

1 cup whipped cream

1 cup milk

2 vanilla pods

10 egg yolks

4 tbsp sugar + extra for topping

Directions:

1. In a pan, add the milk and whipped cream. Cut the vanilla pods open and scrape the seeds into the pan along with the pods.

2. Place the pan over medium heat on a stovetop until almost boiled, stirring regularly.

3. Turn off the heat. Beat egg yolks in a bowl and whisk in sugar, but not too bubbly. Remove the vanilla pods from the milk mixture; pour the mixture onto the egg mixture, stirring constantly.

4. Let rest for 15 minutes. Fill 4 ramekins with the mixture and cover tightly with foil. Place them in the frying basket and Bake at 170 F for 25 minutes.

5.Remove the ramekins and discard the foil; let cool at room temperature, then refrigerate for 1 hour.

6.Sprinkle the remaining sugar over the crème brûlée and use a torch to caramelize the top. Serve immediately or chilled. Enjoy!

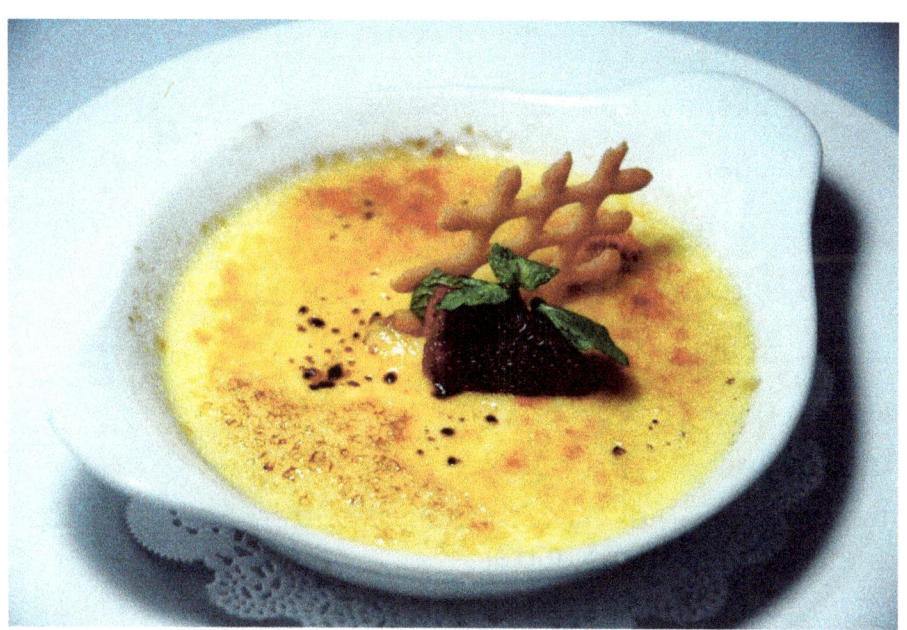

White Chocolate Pudding

Cook Time:

30 minutes

Servings: 4

Ingredients:

3 oz white chocolate

4 egg whites

2 egg yolks, at room temperature

¼ cup sugar

1 tbsp melted butter

1 tbsp cold butter

¼ tsp vanilla extract 1

½ tbsp flour

Directions:

1. Coat two ramekins with melted butter. Swirl in 2 tbsp of sugar to coat the butter.

2. Melt the cold butter with the chocolate in a microwave; set aside. In another bowl, beat the egg yolks vigorously.

3. Add the vanilla and the remaining sugar; beat to incorporate fully. Mix in the melted chocolate. Add the flour and mix until there are no lumps.

4. Preheat air fryer to 330 F. Whisk the egg whites in another bowl until the mixture holds stiff peaks.

5. Fold in the chocolate mixture and divide the mixture between the ramekins. Place them in the frying basket, and Bake for 14-16 minutes, until cooked through. Enjoy!

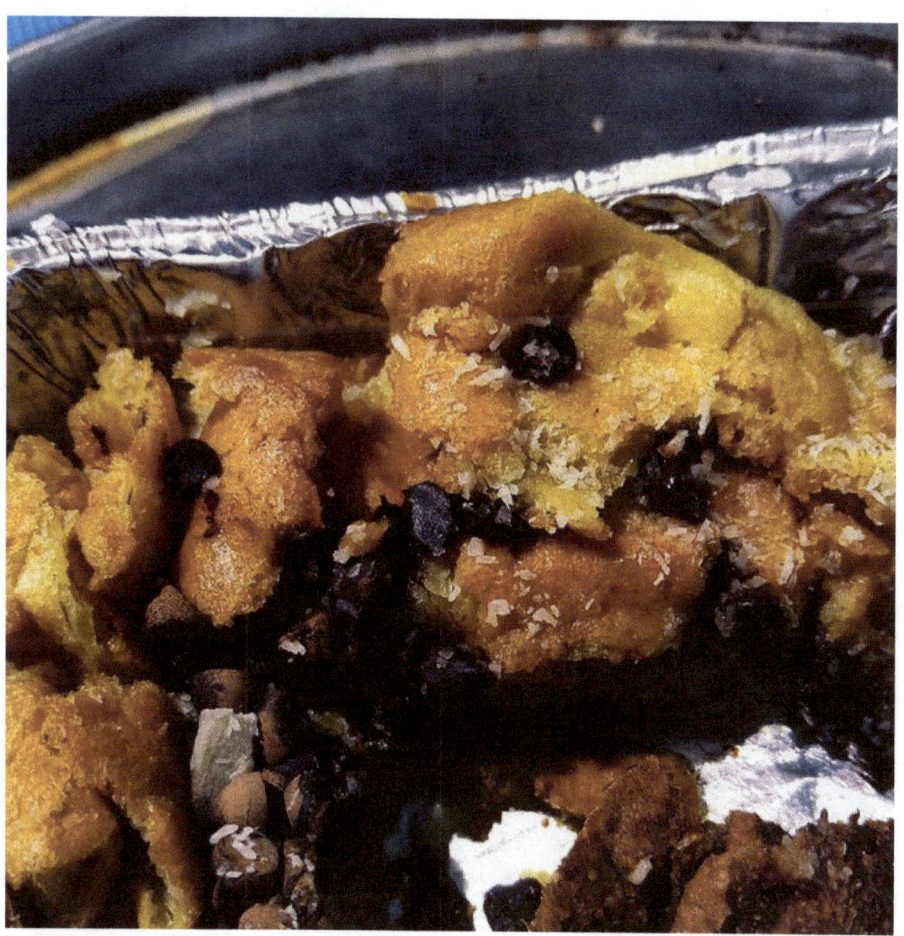

Cinnamon Grilled Pineapples

Cook Time:

30 minutes

Servings: 2

Ingredients:

1 tsp cinnamon

5 pineapple slices

½ cup brown sugar

1 tbsp mint, chopped

1 tbsp honey

Directions:

1. Preheat air fryer to 340 F. In a small bowl, mix sugar and cinnamon. Drizzle the sugar mixture over pineapple slices.

2. Place them in the greased frying basket and Bake for 5 minutes. Flip the pineapples and cook for 5 more minutes. Drizzle with honey and sprinkle with fresh mint. Enjoy!

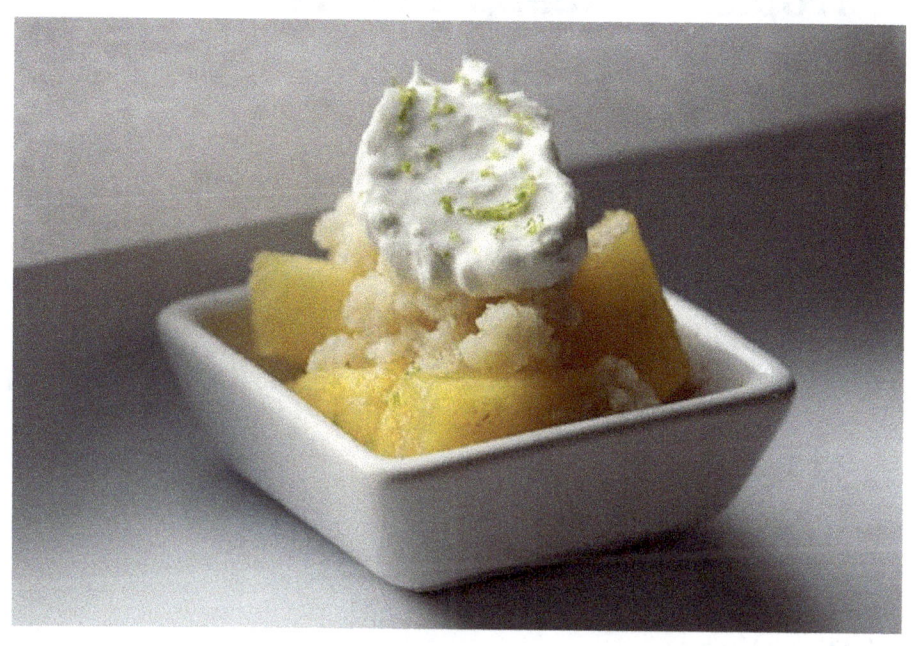

Tropical Pineapple Fritters

Cook Time:

30 minutes

Servings: 5

Ingredients:

1 ½ cups flour

1 pineapple, sliced into rings

3 tbsp sesame seeds

2 eggs, beaten

1 tsp baking powder

½ tbsp sugar

Directions:

1. Preheat air fryer to 350 F. In a bowl, mix salt, sesame seeds, flour, baking powder, eggs, sugar, and 1 cup water.

2. Dip sliced pineapple in the flour mixture and arrange them on the greased frying basket. Air Fryer for 15 minutes, turning once. Enjoy!

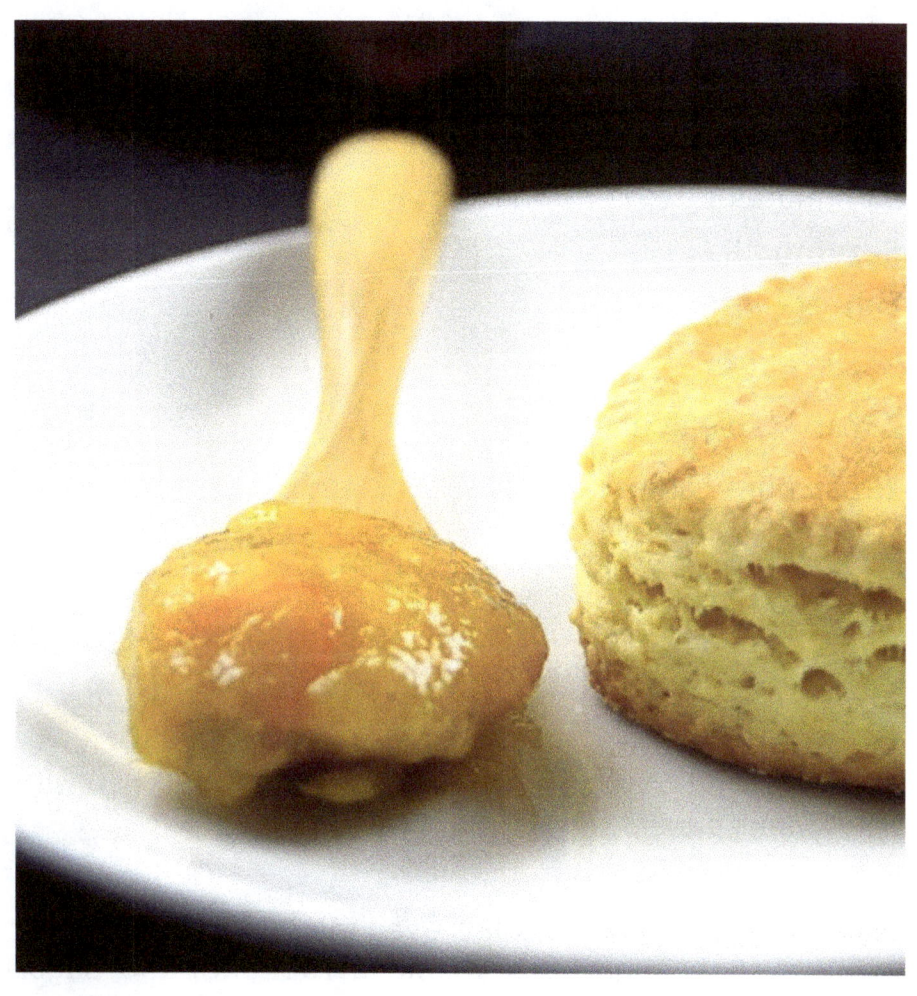

Apricot & Lemon Flapjacks

Cook Time:

30 minutes

Servings: 4

Ingredients:

¼ cup butter

2 tbsp maple syrup

2 tbsp pure cane sugar

1 ¼ cups rolled oats

2 tsp lemon zest

3 apricots, stoned and sliced

DIRECTIONS

1. Preheat air fryer to 350 F. Line a baking dish with parchment paper.

2. Melt the butter in a skillet over medium heat and stir in pure cane sugar and maple syrup until the sugar dissolves, about 2 minutes.

3. Mix in the remaining ingredients and transfer to the baking dish. Bake for 18-20 minutes or until golden. Let cool for a few minutes before cutting into flapjacks Enjoy!

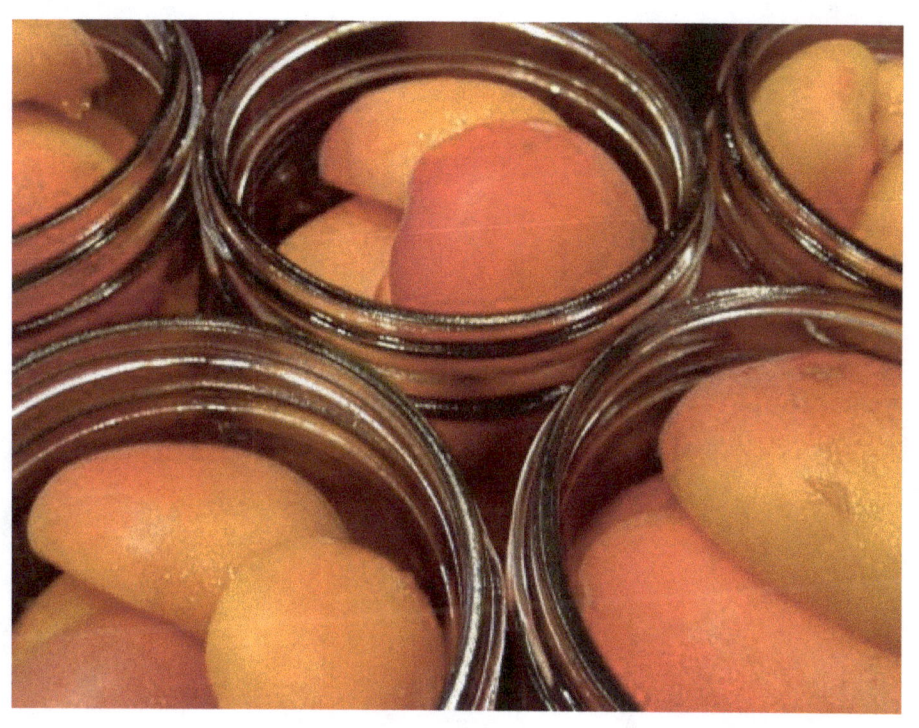

www.ingramcontent.com/pod-product-compliance
Lightning Source LLC
Chambersburg PA
CBHW070725030426
42336CB00013B/1922